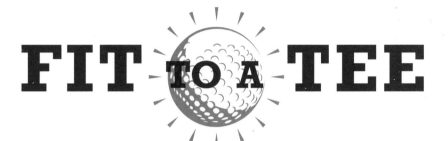

FIT
TO A
TEE

The Ultimate Endurance, Strength & Flexibility System for Golfers of Every Ability

Edward Jackowski, Ph.D.

Foreword by Gary Player

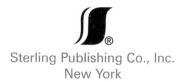

Sterling Publishing Co., Inc.
New York

Dedication

I would like to dedicate this book to my father, who took the time and made the effort to introduce me to the wonderful game of golf, and a myriad of other sports. It wouldn't have been possible for me to achieve my level of athleticism, confidence, and hunger to help coach others without his guidance and input.

I also would like to thank my wife Laura, who was inspirational and patient during the time needed to complete this book project.

Special thanks to Doug, C.J., and Adrian, whose input helped educate me in what type of fitness everyday golfers need to improve their distance and overall golf game.

And to Lawrence, whose special illustration skills and talents made this book complete.

Published by Sterling Publishing Co., Inc.
387 Park Avenue South, New York, NY 10016

© 2007 by Sterling Publishing Co., Inc.

Distributed in Canada by Sterling Publishing
c/o Canadian Manda Group, 165 Dufferin Street,
Toronto, Ontario, Canada M6K 3H6

Distributed in the United Kingdom by GMC Distribution Services,
Castle Place, 166 High Street, Lewes, East Sussex, England BN7 1XU

Distributed in Australia by Capricorn Link (Australia) Pty. Ltd.
P.O. Box 704, Windsor, NSW 2756, Australia

ISBN-13: 978-1-4027-3216-4
ISBN-10: 1-4027-3216-3

Illustrations by
Lawrence Hosannah

Printed in China

2 4 6 8 10 9 7 5 3 1

For information about custom editions, special sales, premium and
corporate purchases, please contact Sterling Special Sales
Department at 800-805-5489 or specialsales@sterlingpub.com.

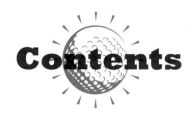

Contents

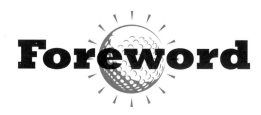

Foreword

I have always been a tremendous advocate of fitness for everyone, whether you play golf, are thinking of playing golf, or have other interests. Golfers of all levels often don't realize how vital it is to have a fit, flexible, and toned body, and how this translates to your golf swing, balance, mental focus, and every other facet of your golf game.

From engaging in a regular fitness regimen, we can strengthen and protect our back, hips, and legs—the places our body experiences the most stress when we play golf. And to thoroughly enjoy golf, as a weekend warrior or recreational golfer, you should condition your body not just for golf, but to improve every other aspect of your active lifestyle.

Being fit has not only allowed me the ability to become better at golf, it has also enabled me to remain mentally and physically focused throughout my career. Even if I have a bad hole, I can bounce back quickly due to my good physical condition. It is the reason I've been able to play golf for so many years without sustaining any major injuries. Being fit has also allowed me to manage my hectic schedule as I've logged over 14 million miles traveling around the world as an international ambassador of golf.

I met Edward at a Champions Tour pro-am tournament and was impressed with his passion for helping people, especially his work with individuals who suffer from diabetes, and his commitment to fitness for golfers, as well as the general public. The fitness regimens Edward has designed are simple to follow, don't require a lot of fancy equipment, are effective, and most important, are safe and easy to follow at all levels of fitness.

So if you want to improve your golf game, hit the ball farther, and extend your golf years, please take the time to educate yourself with *Fit to a Tee*.

GARY PLAYER
Grand Slam Golfer

Introduction

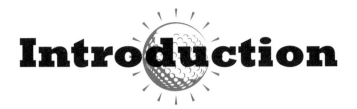

To me, golf is one of the most pleasurable of all leisure activities. It allows you to learn about yourself and challenge yourself. You learn patience, decision-making skills, and how to perform under pressure. You never tire of the thrill of hitting a great drive or sinking a long putt. And, like fitness, you never truly master the game, so it keeps you coming back for more!

I mention these wonderful characteristics of golf because my objective in this book is to prepare you physically and mentally to get the most out of the game. Unlike most sports, you really can't injure yourself too seriously playing golf—unless, of course, you're not physically fit. So, as you read on, please keep in mind that I am your biggest fan. I want you not only to feel good while playing golf, but to learn how to keep challenging yourself.

Growing up on the North Shore of Long Island, New York, I was able to caddie at a number of golf courses in the area. When I was eleven years old, I would walk down to the highway nearby and hitchhike to country clubs such as Cedar Brook, Engineers,

Muttontown, Glen Head, North Shore, and Brookville. The first time I showed up to caddie at Cedar Brook, the caddie master made me wait from 7 a.m. to 2 p.m. before I got my first loop. It was with a "honeymoon" couple, the term in golf for a husband and wife who play together after everyone else has teed off for their morning and early afternoon rounds.

I can still remember that day vividly. First of all, I was barely taller than the two bags I needed to carry on my shoulders for the eighteen holes. Second, both husband and wife were all over the golf course, spraying shots to the left, to the right, and out of bounds. It was also during the 1970s, when a caddie hustled and did anything and everything to please club members and prove himself capable—there were so many of us that each member could take his pick. It was very competitive, and if you expected to continue to have a job as a caddie, you needed to earn a favorable grade at the end of each round from whomever you caddied for that particular day. That way, the caddie master would move you up the "corporate ladder" of caddies. The better the caddie, the less time you needed to wait when you arrived at the golf course in the morning. And if you got out early enough, you could easily caddie thirty-six holes that day and maybe even an extra nine on top of that. All I can say is thank goodness I was fit. My parents prepared me both physically and mentally, and made sure I was not only involved in sports but had a number of vigorous chores to do every day after school as well. I had no problem with the physical challenges of the job.

As the years passed, I became quite good at caddying. I not only learned the ins and outs of every aspect of golf, but also honed my skills at clubbing people properly (*clubbing* is choosing the right golf club to match the golfer's distance for a particular shot or selecting a club that will allow the ball to bounce or land a particular way). I also became very good at reading and judging greens, a critical component for scoring well in golf. I paid attention to the nuances, patterns, and habits of the players—specifically, the physical characteristics that both genders exhibited, good and bad.

My father first taught me to swing a golf club when I was about ten years old and I played here and there until I was about eighteen. Then I was involved in other sports and played golf very sparingly until my late thirties, when I could afford the time to play. Today, I am a recreational golfer. Sure, I'd like to play more often, and, yes, I really enjoy the game of golf, but with other priorities—family

Being fit for golf will improve all aspects of your life

responsibilities and work commitments—I'm not able to do so. I am also realistic when it comes to my golf game. Even though I have the ability and potential to be an excellent golfer, as opposed to just a very good golfer, I don't expect to be a scratch golfer because I don't put in the necessary practice time. I only play fifteen to twenty rounds of golf a year, mostly in the summer and fall, but I am still able to maintain a 10 handicap. Not bad, considering I don't practice much and often it is weeks, sometimes months, between golf rounds.

I have always been fortunate to be able to hit the golf ball a great distance, and I possess tremendous club speed due to my strength and excellent flexibility for a man of my size. It is rewarding knowing that on any given day, no matter how long it has been between practice or golf rounds, I can go out there and not only shoot a decent score, but hit the golf ball with enough distance to get home on a par 5 in two shots (provided I hit my drive semistraight, which is more a function of practice than fitness). It is quite an advantage, especially psychologically, knowing—and more important, believing—that I can get on the green from 150 yards away in the rough using a pitching wedge, when my opponent is hitting with a 5, 6, or 7 iron. This confidence allows me to fare well in tournaments, and because I am fit, the way I exercise carries over to my golf game. It is my insurance policy, especially since I can't practice as much as I would like. I want to share with you the fitness strategies that have helped many of my clients over the years increase their distance and improve their scores. You will also greatly enhance your fitness level, improve your health, and help alleviate some stress.

About ten years ago, I started thinking about writing this very book on fitness and golf. I started to keep notes and gather data from all my experiences, from working as a caddie as a young boy to playing at golf clubs as an adult, observing the way people swing. Wherever I went, from a local charity tournament to the golf range, I would see men and women doing the same things, over and over, that kept them from hitting the ball farther or putting well. So, a few years ago, I tracked down one of the best teaching pros in New York, Doug Mauch from Wheatley Hills Golf Club on Long Island. I called Doug, introduced myself, and asked him if he'd be interested in letting me train him to be fit for golf. I also called a women's pro, C.J. Reeves from Century Country Club in Westchester County, New York. It was important to me that this book pay equal attention to the women who play golf, because, too often, golf books (at least those that are written by men) are not very

helpful or useful to women. To give this book an international flair and a wider perspective, I also consulted Adrian Fryer, one of England's top teaching pros. (I visited Adrian in Manchester and took a lesson from him while I was lecturing in the UK in 2005.) And five years ago, I started to hold clinics and seminars at country clubs and companies to teach people how to hit the golf ball for more distance through proper fitness. I thought it was essential to get feedback from teaching pros like Doug, C.J., and Adrian because they teach golf to a cross-section of players, from children to the elderly—this book's exact audience. They have provided me with insight into what both male and female golfers need to work on physically in order to improve their golf game. The result is a book that is a compilation of many elements and has been written to help you become more fit. Being fit will carry over not only to your everyday golf game, helping you to hit the ball farther and with more control, and to score better, but it will also help you to perform better physically and mentally in all aspects of your life.

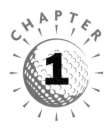

Things You Should Know Before Starting

There are a number of books about exercising to improve your golf game. However, these books don't offer guidelines for how to meet your fitness goals without using a lot of gadgets, complex moves, expensive and technical fitness equipment, or a personal trainer. I have kept the exercise regimens simple so you can maintain consistency with the routines outlined and illustrated in this book. And no golf book—until now—teaches you both how to improve your golf game and how to get in better shape overall. The exercise prescriptions in this book are all you need to improve your health, your fitness, and your golf game. This is a valuable approach because most people can—and will—only devote three to five hours a week to improving their fitness level, even with the best of intentions. Remember, the goal is to be consistent. If you are consistent, you will see results. Generally, it is not you who have failed when a new diet or fitness program does not produce results, but rather the program that has failed you, because it is not compatible with your lifestyle.

Most golfers do not work out with the regularity and intensity necessary to make major improvements in their golf game. It is vital to get a good start with your fitness regimen—not only to perform better on the golf course, but to see improvement in your body as well—and to sustain it. If you find that after working out you are not as tired after a round, or maybe your back is not as achy the next day, that small benefit will help you keep going in pursuit of that nirvana called fitness. Hey, we all want to be better at golf—hit the ball farther, score better—but how many of us are willing to do what it takes to truly achieve these goals?

Many golfers don't have a clue about how to exercise properly to increase their distance and therefore improve their entire golf game. Or they don't realize the importance of being fit, or it just isn't enough of a priority for them. How do you think you're going to hit a golf ball with the same physical power and strength and mental focus on hole No. 18 as you did on hole No. 1 if you're vastly overweight or can't even touch your toes?

Take a look at the men and women who play on all professional levels today. Are they hitting the ball farther because of better equipment or because they are more fit? Let's see. Gone are the days when an overweight, out-of-shape golfer could win more than a few tournaments. If you follow professional golf, you'll see that many more of today's professional golfers are fit, as compared to ten years ago, when fitness was not something commonly observed on the tours. Today, even the out-of-shape golfers of the past have reorganized their priorities and have completely changed their bodies for the better through fitness regimens. That's the main reason why you see so many players over sixty winning senior tournaments and majors!

Take the top ten golfers on all the tours today, add twenty to fifty pounds to their current weight and take away their current fitness regimens. Do you think they would still be in the top ten a year from now? Not a chance! If a professional golfer who hits thousands of balls a week can only slightly improve her game with all the new technology and fitness training, what are the odds that someone who doesn't practice or exercise much at all will increase his distance or improve his golf score? Sure, you may get lucky every once in a while off the tee and hit a bomb (that's the technology working for you, my friend), but you won't significantly improve your everyday golf game unless you commit to getting fit.

According to Doug, C.J., and Adrian, the teaching pros, eight out of every ten people they teach do not even practice the lessons on a regular basis. This brings me to the next important point: a golf pro or swing doctor teaches you how to swing a golf club, correcting your swing flaws, body alignment, posture, and how you address the ball—*period*. So when your pro says, "Bob, you need to turn more" or "Susan, you need to keep your left arm straight when you bring the club back," I don't care if you practice a thousand times a day, you will not be able to do what your pro is asking unless you get yourself physically fit. The ability to turn or keep your left arm straight is more a function of flexibility, range of motion, and strength than technique. If you are struggling in these areas, the only way you will be able to improve is to work on physical conditioning—you have no other options. Only 10 percent of the entire world population exercises three to five days a week. You need to *earn* an improved golf game, by working to develop a fit, toned, and capable body.

What I have learned over the years about human nature by studying people's habits and tendencies in relation to golf and fitness is that we all do want to work out more and practice more, but because of certain lifestyle constraints, it is difficult to do so. I have also found that it is much easier for most people (especially those who live in an urban area) to work out on a regular basis than to hit golf balls at the range, simply because you can exercise

The most important factor in becoming fit is consistency

almost anywhere. If there were a golf range on every block, you certainly would be able to craft your swing a lot better. But would you hit the golf ball with more power and distance? Maybe, but you probably wouldn't see a significant difference. However, if you were to exercise and properly prepare your body for golf and improve your fitness, when you got to a golf range you would be able to practice longer, be more focused, be able to shape your shots more effectively, hit the golf ball farther and with more power, and enjoy the act of "practicing." Yes, being more fit translates over to your golf game in a number of positive ways, including applying what your teacher has drilled into you from day one—whether it is to keep from swaying, to practicing proper follow-through, to not breaking your elbow, to rotating more, or to firing through the ball. That's why I emphasize the importance of working out consistently, properly, safely, efficiently, and effectively, because when your body is fit, it can do anything.

True, golf isn't exactly the most physically demanding sport. Walking the golf course when you play is not a fitness regimen. It is a form of exercise and can be part of your fitness program, but it is only one of the five components that make up the medical meaning of fitness: flexibility, strength, endurance, aerobic capacity, and a healthy body ratio. For golfers, fitness also involves balance, hand-eye coordination, and timing. I know plenty of

people who walk every day yet look like they spend their entire lives at a buffet table in Vegas.

In order to hit a power fade or a controlled draw, as taught to you by your pro, you must possess the power and ability to control your swing. Much of that is based on your flexibility—flexibility affects every aspect of your golf game. This book will teach you—without a golf lesson!—how to add thirty to fifty yards or more to your drive and your other fairway woods and metals, twenty to thirty yards to your iron play, more precision to your putting, and most important, how to gain a renewed confidence in your game. Look, there are many options to choose from if you are trying to exercise for general health, fitness, and golf. But what I want you to learn from this book is to have a plan—a plan that makes you a better player, a plan that makes sense, and one that enables you, the golfer, to become educated and self-reliant, to fine-tune and master proper fitness strategies and incorporate them into your daily life despite any constraint, perceived or real. So sit back and relax, read, learn, and then make a commitment to yourself to become a fitter golfer so that you can truly enjoy your next nine, eighteen, or more holes. Please don't disappoint your Doug, C.J., or Adrian. Start doing something about your fitness level. I promise you, you will surpass all of your golf goals, and your life goals as well.

Why Being Fit Means More Distance

Take a careful look at the golf swings illustrated on the following pages. Although they *look* simple, they involve many muscle groups, large and small, working together to help you achieve maximum performance. You need flexibility and range of motion throughout your body: agility, muscle strength, and endurance in your lower body, midsection (known as your core), and upper body, as well as hand-eye coordination and balance. You also need timing and the ability to stabilize your lower body while turning your upper body, and then moving your lower body slightly as your upper body begins to rotate back toward your target as you power through the ball.

Pretty awesome, huh? Now you can easily see why being fit throughout your entire body lends itself to hitting the golf ball farther consistently, and that with practice and help from your local pro or teacher, you will be able to hit any golf shot with more power and pinpoint accuracy. Want another reason to become fit for golf? Currently, in

the United States alone, there are more than thirty-seven million golfers who want to play better golf, and nearly 80 percent of them will experience some type of pain due to swing faults, poor fitness, or lack of flexibility. A golf swing generates approximately seven times your body weight in compression on the spine and it is one of the most biomechanically complicated movements in all of sports. That's why it's important not only to exercise, but to exercise in a way that boosts your fitness and avoids pain. As a golfer, if you have restricted joints and muscles and lack of flexibility, that reduces your range of motion and causes loss of club speed, additional pain and potential injury, and a decrease in power and balance. As your strength increases (specifically your core and rotational strength), you will see tremendous improvements in your distance and you will not be as sore during and after your round of golf. That means you will play more often and require less recovery time between matches—in general, golfing will be a more positive experience for you as you continue to play. Many golfers spend more money and time looking for that secret gadget to raise their level of play than they spend on the vehicle in which they ride twenty-four hours a day—their bodies!

Golf, unlike most sports, does not allow you to "play your way into shape." Golf is played in the late spring, summer, and early fall, unless you live in a climate that enables you to play year-round. I have noticed that the people who are not able to play year-

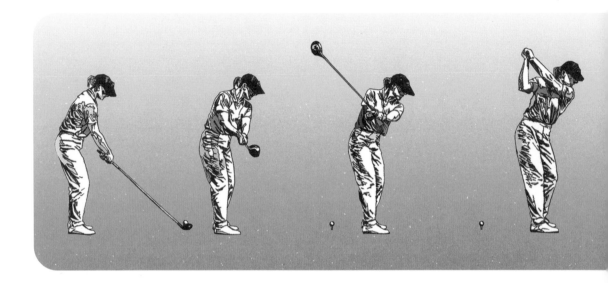

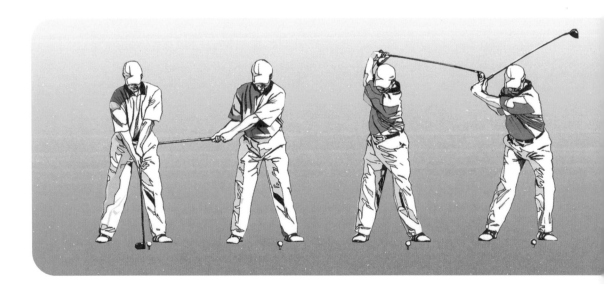

round are in better physical condition than those who can play any day of the year. Why? Perhaps because once you get into the swing of the season, you don't have time for the gym, and if you are able to play year-round, you tend to spend that valuable workout time playing the game instead of combining the two elements. That's why I have included in-season and off-season training and exercise regimens for you to follow.

According to my trio of pros, most men lack physical flexibility—especially in their

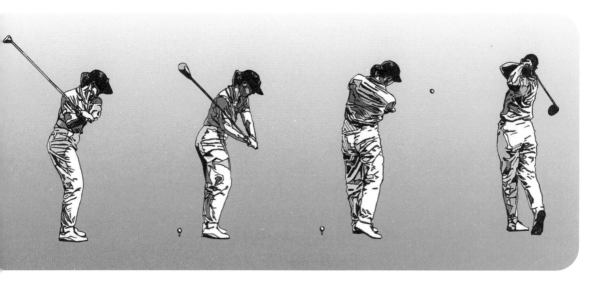

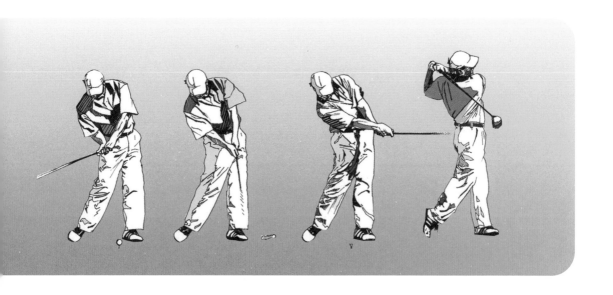

hamstrings (muscles located on the back of each leg) and the upper back and shoulder region—and have weak abdominal and core muscles. Women, on the other hand, generally have much better flexibility, as well as stronger abdominals and core regions, but lack hand, wrist, forearm, arm, and shoulder strength. Deficits in any of these areas prevent you from firing through the ball properly to maximize distance and accuracy. A good golf swing requires three simple moves—shift, turn, and hit—and the distance you hit a golf ball depends on your physical ability to excel in these three simple movements. No matter how competitive or noncompetitive you are when you play golf, there is still mental stress and pressure associated with each shot and putt. Generally, people under pressure don't rise to the occasion; rather, they fall to their level of training. So being fit carries over to your golf swing as well as your golf score, your play under pressure, and all the other mental "games" associated with playing golf at all levels.

Now let's turn to what is needed physiologically to perform a full golf swing and what constitute the basic components associated with most golf shots.

> **A good golf swing requires three simple moves—shift, turn, and hit**

Flexibility

All golf shots, including putting, require optimal flexibility in all joints of the body in order for you to perform a correct swing. Good flexibility helps improve your scoring by allowing you to add distance, precision, and accuracy to each golf shot, and it also prevents injury. Most golfers suffer from inflexibility and imbalances that impede their progress; higher handicappers frequently come "over the top" of the ball, causing weak ball flight and trauma to their bodies. Inflexibility in your hamstrings, hips, and shoulders prevents you from having a smooth and powerful golf swing.

Unless you improve your flexibility, you will never execute a sound swing. In addition to stretching before you engage in your workout regimen, all golfers—men and women alike—should stretch before, during, and after playing, especially those whose flexibility is poor. Depending on where your body is most inflexible, spend a bit more time stretching the tight regions so that those areas can loosen up and become as flexible as your more free-moving regions, making you more balanced throughout your body. Often, when you are playing a round, after the first six holes or so you might hear someone say, "I'm finally warmed up—I'm going to play the back nine better." The truth is, if you warmed up and stretched properly *before* you set out to play, you wouldn't throw away valuable strokes and you'd score better each and every round.

Strength and Endurance

Strength and endurance are essential for a good and powerful golf swing. Yet training for strength and endurance causes the most injuries. While you need to be strong to swing a golf club, golf does not require the same strength as most other sports. It actually requires more endurance in certain muscle groups than pure strength.

Strength is the ability to move a maximum amount of weight one or two times, whereas *endurance* is defined as moving a lighter object many times without the need for rest. But the more times you are able to move a lighter object (such as a golf club) with the same force and power without getting fatigued is a form of strength. That's why, since a golf swing requires strength throughout a full range of motion, it is essential that your exercises mimic and carry over to your golf game. This is called *functional training* because it is necessary to your sport at hand. Good examples of this would be a track runner's or swimmer's conditioning programs. Those athletes would certainly not solely lift weights to enhance their sports performance. Their training would include doing running or drills in the pool to get functionally better at their sport.

Although weightlifting has been a major part of a lot of professional golfers' training regimens, I am not a big proponent of *heavy* weightlifting, for many reasons. First off, it's very complicated and requires a trainer. Second, you can't mimic the same training regimen if you travel. There is also a high risk of serious injury. Lifting heavy weights tends to cause limited range of motion and decrease flexibility, and it puts unwanted bulk on specific areas of our bodies. You really don't need all that strength to hit a golf ball farther—it's overkill.

I do believe, however, in strength training, and if you are lifting weights, I recommend very light to moderate weights with a high number of repetitions. There are more effective ways to train for golf without using traditional weights, as you will see in the chapters ahead. The first rule of thumb when you embark on a fitness regimen—whether it is for golf, general fitness, weight loss, or any other reason—is to maintain the program today, tomorrow, next month, next year, and five years from now. If you can't do that, don't even attempt it, because you will fail. In other words, you may receive an A for effort, but an F for follow-through.

Strengthening your abdominal and core region will help make your swing more efficient, as well as prevent injury. Most golfers try to generate more power and club speed with their shoulders and arms by swinging harder or faster, creating additional trauma to their joints. That kind of swing stresses the lower back, hips, shoulders, and elbows, as compared to a proper swing. Golf is very one-sided, just like tennis, so you need to exercise to counter-balance the stresses to one side of your body. Light dumbbell work, chin-ups, dips, push-ups, and pull-ups are good examples of adding unilateral (using one joint during a movement) and

Fitness is flexibility, strength, endurance, aerobic capacity, and a healthy body ratio

multiplanar (using multiple joints during a movement) capabilities. Having a variety of exercises in your repertoire will boost your fitness and relieve boredom as well.

Many elderly men, at the range or on the golf course, have a quick, jerky, hurried swing. Aside from lacking flexibility, their swing is not balanced, so they lose virtually all their power. And although we do lose strength and flexibility as we age, if we train our bodies properly, we can slow down this process more than we think. The problem for many of these older golfers is that they were never flexible or strong enough even in their prime, so now their bodies age exponentially faster. The good news is that anyone, regardless of age, can greatly improve in all aspects of fitness. So if you do possess this type of swing, it can be corrected, but only through a fitness regimen.

I like most strengthening and endurance exercises to be performed while standing, to help with balance, posture, and stability. Most of your golf swing's power is derived from the torso and lower body musculature. Lower body strength is also essential for improving balance, which is critical throughout the entire golf swing, but particularly at the swing's completion. (See illustrations above right.) I like angled squats, dead lifts, and one-legged step-ups as a few examples for strengthening the lower body. For your core region and abdominals, full bent-knee sit-ups, leg-outs, elbows to knees, and knees to elbows are a few of the exercises I advocate for golfers.

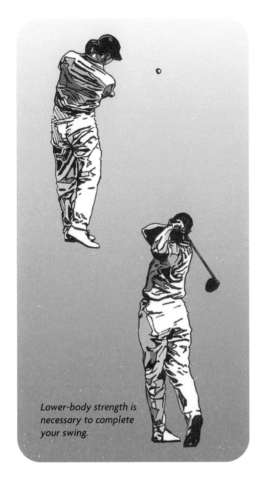

Lower-body strength is necessary to complete your swing.

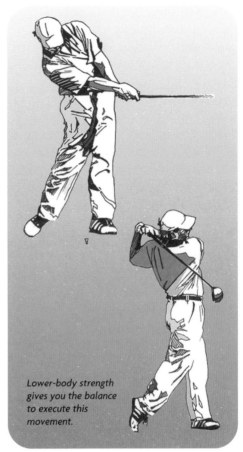

Lower-body strength gives you the balance to execute this movement.

Aerobic Capacity

The good news is that, in theory, you do not need to be very aerobically fit to play golf, unlike other sports, such as basketball or swimming. And if you ride a golf cart more than you walk the golf course, your aerobic capacity does not play as large a role in your fitness as those who walk most of their rounds. If you do walk more than you ride in a golf cart while playing golf, you definitely need to be more aerobically fit, for obvious reasons.

Being aerobically fit has many benefits that carry over to your golf game, other than simply being able to walk a round without feeling fatigued. I have noticed that most people who ride a golf cart are more out of shape and tend to be more overweight than those who walk the course. This is because it requires much more energy to walk and carry your clubs or even use a pushcart for eighteen holes as opposed to just getting in and out of a golf cart.

Improving your aerobic capacity is especially important for golfers who are overweight. In fact, you cannot lose weight unless most of your exercise time is devoted to aerobic training, so if you need to lose weight, be sure to spend more time performing aerobic-type exercises. You will swing more freely and easily by losing weight (your stomach will be smaller, allowing you greater range of motion) and cause less wear and tear on your core region, especially your back—all good reasons to lose weight, along with all the general health benefits associated with weight loss. The best exercises for improving your aerobic capacity and losing weight are jogging, jumping rope, cross-country skiing or using a similar-type machine, and walking at a brisk pace on a golf course or treadmill with different terrains that mimic your golf game. For those who cannot walk fast enough to derive aerobic benefits or who suffer from other medical and/or ortho-pedic problems, a recumbent stationary bike is the best fitness investment you can make because you can pedal at a fast pace (70–100 rpm) with little resistance, which will not stress your knees or back because you are totally supported while performing the exercise.

Another benefit to becoming more aerobically fit is that your heart becomes more efficient, which carries over to the other exercises you will be performing. Hence, your recovery time will be shorter

and you will be able to exercise with more intensity for longer periods. This means you burn more calories each time you work out, increasing your fitness level at a much faster pace. Aerobically fit individuals tend to fatigue less in their lower body, so on a hot day or on very hilly terrain, they make fewer swing mistakes and are able to finish the round without pain or anguish.

Please note: your body ratio is your proportion of lean muscle to body fat, based on your body weight. Like flexibility, strength, endurance, and aerobic capacity, a healthy body ratio is one of the key components of fitness.

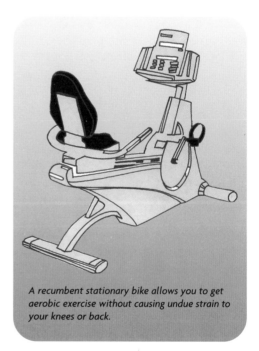

A recumbent stationary bike allows you to get aerobic exercise without causing undue strain to your knees or back.

Performance

The ability to twist your shoulders back while keeping your hips straight, the strength to hold the club in position at the top of the backswing, and the ability to fully extend your arms during the downswing through the ball are just a few examples of the physical elements needed to hit the ball properly. Whether you practice a little or a lot, you will not succeed at hitting the ball farther and more accurately and improving your score unless you have the proper alignment, strength, and flexibility. Balancing exercise time and practice time on the range is important because you do not want to overtrain or overhit, which will cause injury. Recovery time between exercise bouts and rounds differs from individual to individual, and the more fit you become, the less your joints and body will feel the torque and stress. On the other hand, the tighter you are, the more inflexible you are, and the more medical or orthopedic concerns you have, the more time you will need to recover. I suggest that unfit golfers swing no more than forty to fifty full swings a day for practice, semifit individuals no more than fifty to seventy swings daily, and very fit individuals about eighty to one hundred full swings a day. After that, your swing usually starts to break down and you start to overcompensate, leading to possible injuries.

Are You Fit Enough for Golf?

A simple fitness test follows to help you figure out which areas of fitness you need to focus on as you begin to exercise for golf: flexibility, strength, endurance, aerobic capacity, balance, hand-eye coordination, or timing.

Judge yourself based on the illustration for each stretch or refer to the DVD, and give yourself a fair rating based on how far you can stretch compared to the illustration. Then, a point value is given for a repetition range within each of twelve categories: upper body flexibility, core flexibility, lower body flexibility, upper body strength, core strength, lower body strength, upper body endurance, core endurance, lower body endurance, aerobic capacity, balance, and hand-eye coordination and timing. Add the points together, based on your current workout routine, to evaluate your golf fitness. For example, a man who does 7 to 9 chin-ups would add the number 3, which is average; a man who does 13+ would add a 5, an excellent score. The top total score is 60 points.

Fitness Test

Hardly Any or None—1 Poor—2 Average—3 Good—4 Excellent—5
*Please refer to the DVD to view these moves.

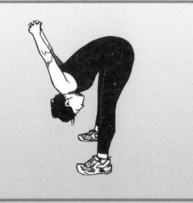

Upper Body Flexibility for Men and Women*

Upper body stretch

Grasp your hands behind your back, with palms facing each other. Slightly bend your knees and lift your arms up as you bend forward at the waist. Hold when you feel a comfortable stretch in the shoulders and chest. Exhale at the furthest point in the stretch.

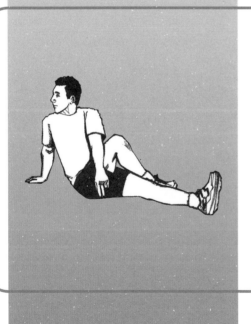

Core Flexibility for Men and Women*

Torso stretch

Sitting on the ground, keep your left leg straight, right arm behind you for support. Cross your right leg over your left knee and place your right foot outside your left knee. With the left hand or elbow on the right knee or thigh, slowly twist, and look over your right shoulder while simultaneously pulling the right knee in the opposite direction; hold. Exhale at the furthest point in the stretch. You will feel pressure in the hip, side, and back. Repeat on the opposite side.

Lower Body Flexibility for Men and Women*

Hamstring stretches

Bend over and place your hands out in front of you on the ground with your legs straight. Flex your ankles and lean back on your heels while balancing yourself on your fingers. Or sit down on the ground with your legs straight, ankles flexed. Bend forward from your hips and grab your toes and hold the stretch. Keep your breathing as steady as possible.

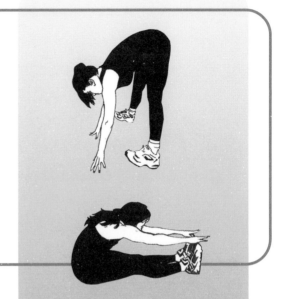

Upper Body Strength for Men

Chin-ups

Hold the bar with your palms facing you about 6 inches apart. Pull yourself up as you exhale, trying to get your chin at or above the bar. Then lower yourself as you inhale until your arms are straight and you're back at the starting position.

0–3 repetitions—1
4–6 repetitions—2
7–9 repetitions—3
10–12 repetitions—4
13+ repetitions—5

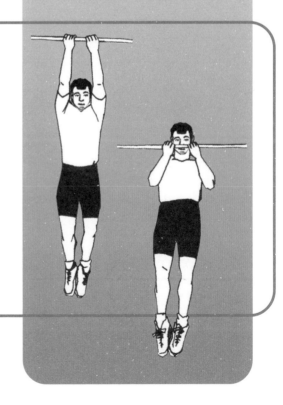

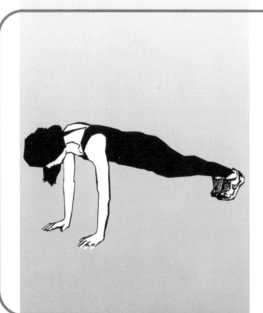

Upper Body Strength for Women

Push-ups on toes

Extend your body on your hands and toes, with your arms straight, and place your hands farther than shoulder-width apart, your fingers forward and abdominals contracted. While inhaling, lower your body toward the floor and lightly touch your chest. Exhale while pushing up to the starting position and repeat. Do not arch your back or jerk your body.

0–3 repetitions—1
4–7 repetitions—2
8–11 repetitions—3
12–15 repetitions—4
16+ repetitions—5

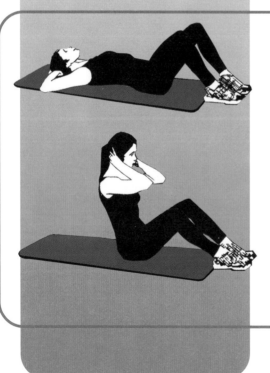

Core Strength for Men and Women

Advanced sit-ups

Lie on your back with your knees bent, feet flat on the floor, heels up against your mat, and your hands on your ears, as shown. Slowly raise your body all the way up, bringing your elbows toward your knees. Exhale while sitting up. Slowly lower your body to the starting position as you inhale, and repeat.

0–5 repetitions—1
6–14 repetitions—2
15–25 repetitions—3
26–35 repetitions—4
36+ repetitions—5

Lower Body Strength for Men and Women

Leg lifts

Lie on your back on the mat with your body fully extended, your hands palms down under or next to your buttocks, as shown, your feet 3 to 8 inches off the ground. Keeping your legs straight and your knees locked, raise your legs to a 90-degree angle. Lower your legs, keeping them as straight as possible and repeat. Exhale as you bring your legs up and inhale as you lower them back toward the floor. Do not arch your back.

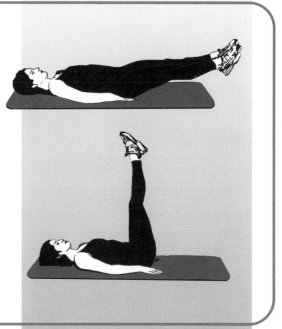

0–3 repetitions—1   *15–22 repetitions—4*
4–8 repetitions—2   *23+ repetitions—5*
9–14 repetitions—3

Upper Body Endurance for Men and Women

Front press with weighted bar
(15–20-lb. for men, 8–10-lb. for women)

Keep your back straight, knees slightly bent, and feet hip-width apart. Grip the bar just past shoulder width and rest the bar across the top of your chest. Fully extend your arms upward and raise the bar straight up while exhaling. Bend your arms and slowly return the bar to the top of your chest while inhaling and repeat.

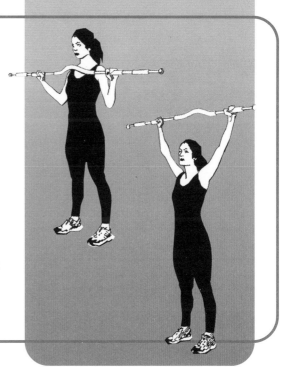

0–10 repetitions—1   *30–39 repetitions—4*
11–19 repetitions—2   *40+ repetitions—5*
20–29 repetitions—3

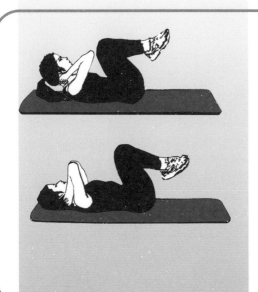

Core Endurance for Men and Women

Elbows to knees

Lying on your back, raise your knees and feet toward your chest in a tucked position. Clasp your hands at the base of your neck. Gently curl your upper body, bringing your elbows toward your knees while exhaling. Slowly lower your back and shoulders to the mat while inhaling and repeat. Keep your lower body motionless.

0–10 repetitions—1   30–39 repetitions—4
11–19 repetitions—2   40+ repetitions—5
20–29 repetitions—3

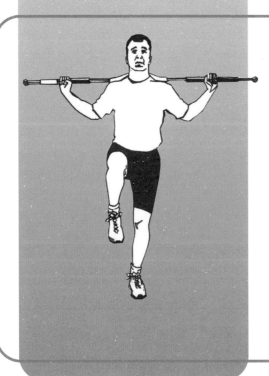

Lower Body Endurance for Men and Women

March in place on toes with aerobic bar

Rest the aerobic bar across your shoulders with your feet hip-width apart and balance yourself up on your toes. Raise your left knee straight up to waist level, aiming toward your chest. Keep your back straight and your abdominals contracted. Lower your left foot to the starting position and switch to raising your right knee. Alternate legs rhythmically. While marching in place, try to stay up on your toes—try not to let your heels touch the ground at any time.

0–25 repetitions—1   60–79 repetitions—4
26–40 repetitions—2   80+ repetitions—5
41–59 repetitions—3

Aerobic Capacity for Men and Women

Jump rope or jogging

Jump Rope

0–2 minutes—1   7–10 minutes—4
2–4 minutes—2   10+ minutes—5
4–7 minutes—3

Jogging at 6 mph, flat surface with no incline or hills

0–1 mile—1   3–4 miles—4
1–2 miles—2   4+ miles—5
2–3 miles—3

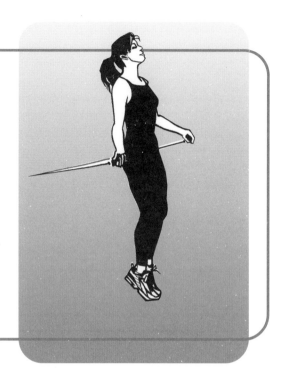

Balance

Stand on one leg with opposite leg bent at waist level and arms out at 90-degree angles.

0–30 seconds—1   2–3 minutes—4
30–60 seconds—2   3+ minutes—5
1–2 minutes—3

Hand-Eye Coordination and Timing

Catch a tennis ball with one hand (not your dominant hand) standing 8 feet away from someone who throws at eye level.

Catches in a row, without dropping

0–3 catches—1   13–17 catches—4
4–7 catches—2   18+ catches—5
8–12 catches—3

Ratings

1–12	What are you waiting for?
13–24	Try harder, you need improvement.
25–36	Not bad, not bad . . . that's a C.
37–48	Nothing wrong with this score.
50–60	Great, now get to the range and practice.

So, how did you do?

Remember, this is just a guide, and although you may rate very well in some areas and poorly in others, it is better to rate well in all areas—it is overall fitness that will allow you to use your particular strong points to your best advantage. For instance, you may possess great strength throughout your body but lack flexibility; as a result, your limited range of motion allows you to utilize only a fraction of your overall body strength in your swing. Or you may have great flexibility, but poor balance or hand-eye coordination so, again, your flexibility is not necessarily helping you swing better.

It's also important to mention that you may be highly flexible in a static state (when you are not moving), but that does not necessarily mean that you have such ability when you are in motion. If this is the case, you don't have the range of motion necessary to achieve greater club speed and power as you swing. For example, consider a woman who normally possesses great upper body and shoulder flexibility while she's stretching, yet cannot keep her left arm perfectly straight when drawing the club back during her backswing because her arms and shoulders are either weak or simply are not used to the range of motion needed for the backswing. This flexibility, then, does not translate into power. (For a lefty golfer, the right arm needs to remain straight.)

> ## Bonus: Mental Toughness
>
> This is easy to gauge and judge yourself on. Basically, you want to take into consideration how hard you exercise, if and when you do, whether you're a passive exerciser or an aggressive exerciser, and whether you strive to do more or do only the minimum. If you've never exercised before on a regular basis, then give yourself a score of 1.

Now it's time to choose what you want out of your fitness regimen, based on your goals. Your goals should be primarily geared toward your weak areas. Most people, when they do exercise, spend the majority of their exercise time doing what they are good at because it is easy and it is within their comfort zone. That's why it's rare for people to reach their fitness goals. Once you have reviewed the Fitness Test and Ratings Scale, choose the exercise regimens associated with bettering your weak areas of fitness.

The following two chapters will help you organize your exercise time, and guide you in performing your workout regimen efficiently, safely, and effectively.

Preparing Yourself for Exercise

The actual act of exercising is not all that difficult. Think about it—you put on some workout clothes, break a sweat for about an hour or so, and poof, you're finished. What's more arduous is organizing your day-to-day activities so that you can exercise consistently. This chapter is your guide to maintaining consistency. It doesn't matter how effective or amazing the exercise regimen is; if you can't follow it regularly, you will never increase your fitness level enough to hit the golf ball farther and with more control. Keep in mind that consistency is the most important element of any fitness regimen.

Get a Physical

If you are over twenty-five years of age and are not exercising vigorously at this time, you should get a full physical as well as a stress test before starting a new exercise program—no exceptions! I'm shocked every time someone who is about to begin an exercise program tells me she has not had a full physical for years. There are many sound reasons for getting a physical, but the best way for me to motivate those who don't regularly receive a check-up is by giving them a reality check: God forbid you develop a disease or condition that you're not aware of, and it festers or lingers within your body for years without attention. The chances of survival are slim at best. But, had you received a physical each year, you would be able to address and treat any problem that arises immediately, and chances are you'd make a full recovery. So please, get a physical. You can never be too safe or too sure.

The other reason to get a physical, especially if you've been sedentary, is to consult your doctor about the intensity at which you should begin exercising. Even if you're in "good health," your heart rate is not used to jumping from your standing pulse to the upper portion of your training zone. This is especially true for former athletes, who were once in fine shape but for the last ten years have been sitting at a desk, or have a lot of stress in their lives. You cannot and should not start exercising where you last left off ten years ago; it will put you at high risk for injury or even the possibility of a heart attack. So, if you have not performed a full body exercise routine with any kind of regularity lately, please start out slowly. Within a few short weeks, you'll be able to increase your intensity and the duration of your workouts. And if you have a special medical problem, seek professional help before you begin to exercise so that you do not exacerbate your condition.

Assess Your Lifestyle

This section is designed to educate and motivate you to perform your workouts in whatever environment you find yourself. From time to time, your schedule will change and life will throw you a curveball that will disrupt your day-to-day routine. Anticipating and preparing for certain lifestyle constraints will allow you to complete your workouts on a consistent basis. Assessing your lifestyle will help you choose where, when, and for how long you need to be exercising to reach your goals. You need to look at your lifestyle and address your particular situation so that you can ultimately be successful. This is as important as determining and following your workout regimen. You will be more successful in getting fit if you organize and prioritize your life so that working out becomes a habit, not an afterthought. If you are just starting out and don't already have a specified workout place or dedicated exercise time slot, or you're not consistent with your workouts, you need to ask yourself these questions:

- Do you work? What are your hours?
- Do you commute?
- Do you travel often for work or pleasure?
- Do you have a gym membership and can you get there on a consistent basis?
- Do you have a gym in the building or complex where you live or at your golf club, and are its hours convenient?
- Do you have young (preteen) children? If so, do you have help (i.e., a nanny, husband, wife) who can supervise them while you're exercising?

These questions will help determine where you should be exercising, how many and which days you'll be working out, and how long you can devote to each workout.

The workouts I'm recommending do not require a lot of fitness equipment or space, so if you travel often, all you need to do is make sure that the hotel where you will be staying has a stationary bike or treadmill; the rest you'll be able to take with you. And even if your location has no fitness equipment, you can still walk, jog, run, or jump rope to get in your aerobic component.

You only need an hour, three to five days a week, to devote to your workouts. If you cannot afford that much time, you can split up your workouts into two half-hour time slots, but I'd prefer you do it all at once—it will be less of a hassle for you. But if you don't have any alternative, then you need to do whatever it takes in order to be consistent with your fitness regimen. If you currently belong to a gym or health club, or are thinking of joining one, there are a few things to consider: if it takes more than fifteen to twenty minutes to get there either by walking or by car, don't join, unless you have a very relaxed schedule and virtually no responsibilities other than taking care of yourself. That one-hour workout just turned into a minimum two-hour commitment: twenty minutes to get there, sixty minutes to exercise, twenty minutes to shower, and twenty minutes to get home. Most people do not have two hours a day to allocate to their fitness. That's one of the reasons why, statistically, only two out of ten people who join a health club or gym utilize it twice a week. The minute a stressor or change in your personal or professional life occurs, the first thing that usually suffers is your workouts. If you find yourself in this predicament, and you really enjoy going to the gym, then you need to get some fitness equipment at home so that when you can't get to your health club, you can exercise at home. So before you join any gym or health club, make sure you can get there under any circumstances; otherwise, choose to exercise at home or, if you can afford it, at both the gym and at home.

I'm often asked, "Is it better to work out in the morning or the evening?" There is not a lot of medical evidence to support either side. The best time for you to be exercising is whenever your schedule allows you to exercise for forty-five to sixty minutes without interruption. Try to choose a time, preferably the same time, to exercise each day. The reason for this is to let your body get used to moving, just as your body is accustomed to eating and sleeping at similar times during the course of a twenty-four-hour period. It's difficult at times to match your preferred time frame with your hectic schedule, but over time, your body will adjust and become used to exercising at that time.

I have found that when I perform high-intensity anaerobic exercises, such as chin-ups, dips, or push-ups in the early morning, I feel tired throughout the day. But when I perform aerobic exercise, such as biking or jumping rope right after I wake up, I feel energized throughout the day. I believe this is because your body and heart rate right after sleeping all night have not had enough time to warm up, and it's a shock to your system when you perform anaerobic-type exercises. During anaerobic exercises, your heart rate soars considerably higher than when you are doing aerobic exercises. So if you need to work out in the early morning and will be doing any type of anaerobic exercises, a longer warm-up will help your body handle your workouts. When you play an early morning round of golf and you are not used to doing so, you'll notice that it takes you a bit longer to get completely warmed up because it feels like your body is still sleeping.

On those days when you have a very early tee-off time, make sure you do a warm-up and then stretch before you take

> **Choose a time, preferably the same time, to exercise each day**

some practice swings or hit balls at the range. You'll see an immediate and rewarding change in your hitting and scoring. And for those of you who must split up your workout—doing some in the morning and some in the evening—try to do your aerobic portion in the morning and your anaerobic portion in the evening.

Sometimes, at the end of your workday, you'll find yourself exhausted, and the last thing you want to do is work out. In fact, you start negotiating with yourself as to whether you're going to make it to the gym. First, you need to ask yourself if your fatigue is due to mental or physical stress. If you had a good night's sleep and had a very grueling day at work, your stress is probably mental, and you should work out as vigorously as possible. But if you had very little sleep, it's physical; you should only do light exercise because in that case you are more at risk of injuring yourself during your workout. If you're tired and don't want to exercise, just tell yourself to get on that bike or treadmill. Once you start moving and break a sweat, your body will begin to wake up and you'll become more alert. Before you know it, you'll be into your workout. This is a learned trait. You need to remind yourself each time you're tired and don't feel like working out that the last time you felt tired, you felt better after you worked out. Focus on just getting on that bike or treadmill and you'll be on your way to maintaining consistency!

When all is said and done, finding time to exercise boils down to priorities. How important is it to you? How much do you want to truly improve your fitness level and better your golf game—to hit the golf ball with more power, distance, and consistency? You must value fitness, just as you value your job enough to show up each day and perform. Are you willing to "sacrifice" some of your idle time and apply it constructively? And here's a good motivator to help you exercise consistently: you'll have the body you desire. The more you see your body change for the better, the more time you will find for fitness. By exercising toward a goal, you will improve your body and the way it functions, and you will be motivated to exercise to stay fit for the rest of your life.

Consider Medical and Orthopedic Constraints

Your medical and orthopedic background dictates what not to do while exercising. In fact, this factor takes precedence over all others when choosing the type of exercises you will be performing. For instance, if you have a severe disc problem in your lower back, even though running may be an effective exercise to lose weight and improve your aerobic capacity, it may not be a wise choice for you. You would be better off utilizing a recumbent stationary bike—which would protect your back—as your primary aerobic activity.

Too often, people either do not go to a specialist for exercise do's and don'ts prior to engaging in a fitness regimen, or they have a precondition and ignore it, thinking that it will go away in time. Remember, if you're injured, you cannot exercise regularly. And if you cannot exercise on a consistent basis, you will barely be able to maintain your current fitness level. You won't be able to properly strengthen and condition your body to play golf more often, and you will not be able to practice more at the range. In order to keep realizing the many benefits that proper exercise and fitness can offer, be smart and exercise your body in a way that does not exacerbate any injury you may have.

Fear of injuring yourself is the number one reason elderly people do not exercise. But having a bad back, leg, or hip is not a sufficient excuse to not exercise. In fact, it is more of a reason to exercise, especially if you ever want to get well and be productive, much less be healthy enough to play—and more importantly—enjoy your golf game. Aside from the health benefits, fitness enables us to enjoy our lives more and become more physically active. Do whatever it takes to get moving.

In all my years in this field, I never once met an individual who did not benefit from proper and regular exercise. With time and perseverance, you will start to increase intensity and be able to add exercises to your regimen that you once thought were impossible. Sometimes we need to walk before we can run. Just because you cannot do every exercise you want from day one, don't use that as an excuse to keep from working out in a way that will eventually yield results.

Here's a good rule to follow while exercising: if it hurts, stop immediately! If you are unable to get advice about a particular exercise and the effect it will have on your body, perform a few repetitions or do a few minutes at a low intensity. That way, if you do exacerbate your condition, you won't do serious or permanent damage to your body. If it feels okay after a day of rest, continue to exercise and slowly begin to increase intensity or duration.

There are many factors that determine how your body will react to an exercise, such as how active you were as a child, how many years you've been exercising, how intensely you exercise, your flexibility, and your mental toughness. If you exercised a certain way for years and now have a medical or orthopedic constraint, the key to maintaining your fitness level and mental stimulation is to substitute that particular exercise with another that will not stress your injured area. For instance, I would like to run more, but growing up, I suffered a number of ankle and leg fractures. So instead of running three to four days a week and stressing my body, I jump rope instead. When my body feels strong, I occasionally run, but never more than one day a week because I know that it will put undue stress on my body and then I will have to rest for days without performing any lower body exercises. In other words, the risk isn't worth the benefit. For those of you who are starting an exercise regimen with aches and pains, especially lower body constraints, I have found that for most people the recumbent stationary bike is the most effective and least stressful to the joints.

Try to work out a minimum of three times a week

Determine Your Current Fitness Level

How hard you're working during your workout is one of the most important factors in determining the success or failure of your fitness program. There are a number of ways to gauge the intensity of your exercise sessions. What's equally important is how to safely increase the intensity of your workouts on a continuous basis. During exercises, your level of intensity can be measured a number of ways: your heart rate during exercise; whether or not you can speak comfortably during aerobic exercise; whether you experience shortness of breath while exercising; or whether you experience dizziness, nausea, muscle fatigue, and chest pains.

Many people do not improve their fitness level and fail to reach their weight loss or fitness goals because they're not exercising with the proper intensity. Calculating your intensity is not an easy task. For instance, you could be working hard enough, but maybe you have chosen the wrong exercises or you're working out too infrequently. There is a lot of controversy over what each individual's intensity level should be during exercise. One thing is for sure, though—if you choose the correct exercises based on your goals, and maintain consistency and intensity, you cannot fail to reach your goals. The easiest way for you to measure intensity is to check your heart rate during a fitness session. The number of heartbeats per minute is one way to monitor your intensity.

As your fitness level improves, your number of heartbeats per minute at rest decreases and you will be able to increase your target heart rate because you will be able to put more strain on your heart

without overdoing it. The more fit you become, the stronger your heart becomes. Even as you age into your sixties, seventies, and eighties, your heart will get stronger if you exercise consistently and properly. However, as your age increases, the recommended number of heartbeats per minute during exercise decreases because you do not want to strain your heart. That doesn't mean that as you age you cannot increase your intensity or fitness level. Your target heart rate (THR) is defined as the heart rate recommended for exercising. When you're in your target heart rate zone, it means you're exercising just vigorously enough. Exercising above your THR means you're exercising too vigorously (out of your zone), and exercising below your THR is referred to as under your zone (not exercising vigorously enough).

How hard should you work during exercise? The amount of energy you expend during exercise (intensity) is the overload you place on your cardiorespiratory system and your entire body during a workout. The threshold needed to achieve benefits is lower for those who are very sedentary compared to those who are very fit. Other factors, such as age, primary risk factors (smoking, heart disease, high blood pressure), and secondary risk factors (over forty-five years of age, family history of heart disease, very stressful lifestyle) dictate how hard you should work out when starting an exercise program.

How your heart will react when you begin an exercise program or add new exercises to your current routine has a lot to do with your current level of fitness.

The risk of sedentary people having heart problems is always higher than it is for those who are more active, because the more active you are, the more your heart is "used" to being taxed. So if you're not active, how much should you push yourself? Most active people are somewhat fit because they need a certain amount of fitness in order to maintain their activity level. That's not to say that they couldn't be a lot more fit, but at least their heart knows the difference when the body goes into motion.

People have a tendency to begin an exercise program either under or over their zone, and very few of them warm up or stretch prior to increasing the intensity (energy) level. Your heart rate increases faster when you're performing anaerobic as opposed to aerobic exercise. A good way to judge how hard you should be exercising is to see how high your heart rate is during the activity, since heart rate increases when intensity increases. To determine your maximal heart rate zone, follow these steps: first estimate what your maximal heart rate should be while exercising. Take the number 220 and subtract your age in years. This number represents your maximal heart rate. For example, a forty-year-old's maximal heart rate would be 180 (220 − 40 = 180). This number means that during any type of physical activity or exercise, your heart rate should not exceed 180 beats per minute. (There are exceptions to this—a well-trained athlete or certain professional athletes who have worked up to this level of intensity, for instance.) You should monitor your heart rate during your exercise period in order to avoid going over your zone and overexerting yourself.

Now that you have figured out your maximal heart rate, the second step to determine your zone is to choose your goals based on how active you are now and your current fitness level. If you cannot accurately determine your current fitness level, assume that you're not as fit as you think and be conservative.

Let's assume that you're an active, semifit forty-year-old whose goal is to lose weight. To calculate 60 percent of your maximal heart rate, which is considered the low end of your zone, you would multiply your maximal heart rate by 60 percent: 180 x 0.60 = 108. That means that in order to gain both fitness and aesthetic benefits from your exercise, you must work hard enough during the exercise for your heart to beat at least 108 beats per minute.

Next, calculate 75 percent of your maximal heart rate to determine the high end of your zone: 180 x 0.75 = 135. So, a forty-year-old semifit woman whose goal is to lose weight should be exercising just hard enough for her heart to beat between 108 and 135 beats per minute. This is exercising in your target heart rate zone.

When beginning an exercise program, make sure you're exercising so that your heart rate is toward the low end of your heart rate zone. I strongly recommend that people over thirty-five years of age take a stress test (EKG, ECG) prior to engaging in any exercise or activity that causes their heart rate to go from a standing pulse (resting heart rate) to 70 percent of their

Figure out your target heart rate (THR) to determine the intensity of your workouts

maximal heart rate. This includes most activities, including walking the golf course.

When starting out, it's more important and safer to increase the time you exercise (duration) than to increase your intensity. Engage in low-intensity exercises, such as riding a stationary bike with light resistance, walking slowly on a treadmill, or taking a beginner exercise class.

Remember to monitor your progress. To determine your heart rate during exercise, find your pulse on your neck or wrist. You can also purchase a heart rate monitor, which shows your heart rate while exercising. Please note that this is highly recommended for people who have any sort of heart condition or who are taking medication that affects their heart rate. Wearing a heart rate monitor will easily allow you to see if you are about to go above your zone, in which case you can immediately lower your intensity or stop. If you're just starting to exercise, remember that the more risk factors you have, the more critical it is for you to exercise closer to the low end or even under the low end of your training zone. Your zone is a range; it's only a guide to follow. If you are exercising and find that you're huffing and puffing, check your pulse. If you are still under your zone, decrease the intensity level immediately. Even though you're under your prescribed zone, you are still deriving benefits from the exercise. In time, you will be able to exercise comfortably within your zone, and eventually you'll be able to increase the intensity of your workouts.

Don't get discouraged if you have to decrease your intensity level. Remaining in your zone during your workout doesn't necessarily mean that you are becoming more fit or that your body will make the desired changes. You could be doing the wrong type of exercises based on your goals. For example, if you are bottom-heavy and are using spinning classes as your primary means of aerobic exercise, you'll never take weight off in that region of your body to your satisfaction, even though you are exercising in your THR zone. Sure, you'll become a little more toned and fit, but you need to be doing different exercises to decrease the size of your lower body.

For those of you thinking of getting a maximum stress test, be careful! (A maximum stress test diagnoses the presence and/or extent of coronary heart disease, in addition to evaluating a person's ability to perform work. By monitoring oxygen consumption during exercise on a treadmill, you are pushed to achieve your maximum work effort. This test can determine cardio-respiratory endurance, as well as whether you have any heart abnormalities. This test should only be performed by highly trained personnel in a clinical setting.) I'm not a big believer in testing sedentary people to find their maximum heart rate, or even 85 percent of their max. Too many things can go wrong. I recommend that those beginning a fitness program purchase a stationary bike and start out cycling at 40 to 60 rpm, with little to no tension or resistance. Your heart rate will not shoot up as fast as it would if you were jogging. Ride for five minutes and take your pulse. Then increase or decrease the speed, noting how you feel and how close you are to your target heart rate zone. If you are comfortable and below your zone, increase the time (duration) by two to five minutes a week and the speed to 60 to 80 rpm, working up to a half-hour or more. When you can cycle for half an hour at 60 to 80 rpm, then start to increase the tension or resistance slightly. This increase in your workload will challenge your aerobic capacity while burning more calories.

Before you start to exercise more intensely, make sure that you've warmed up and stretched properly, especially when performing high-intensity exercises such as push-ups (anaerobic). When you perform push-ups, you're using many smaller muscle groups (i.e., arms, back, chest, and shoulders), which is why you can only do them for a short time. Also, doing push-ups raises your heart rate very quickly, and it does not stabilize at a low enough level for you to take in sufficient oxygen to sustain the exercise. Conversely, jogging, walking, or swimming utilizes larger muscle groups (i.e., legs) and can be sustained for a longer period because your heart rate does not rise as quickly and stays relatively steady during the duration of exercising, allowing you to take in more oxygen. One of the key elements in determining what truly distinguishes aerobic from anaerobic exercise is your heart rate while performing an exercise. Very few people can perform anaerobic exercise at 100 percent of their estimated maximal heart rate for long periods of time unless they are in great physical condition.

Try to perform aerobic exercises that "agree with" your body. Because you will be performing aerobic, as opposed to other, exercise for longer periods of time, it is critical that you are somewhat comfortable while in motion. If you do not like to jog, don't go out and buy a treadmill just because your best pal loves his. Decide with your head what you will enjoy doing when it comes to improving your cardiovascular conditioning.

If you have suffered a heart attack, it is imperative for you to be under a healthcare professional or doctor's care and for you to monitor your heart rate during exercise. For heart attack patients, I highly recommend wearing a heart rate monitor while exercising. It can alert you if you are nearing your maximum heart rate (220 minus your age), as well as help you to stay in your zone while exercising after a heart attack. Remember, each person's body is unique and will react differently while working out. Only your doctor, ideally the doctor who has been treating you for your heart condition, has the most accurate knowledge regarding these and other factors to consider when you are about to embark on an exercise program.

Take Your Heart Rate During Exercise

To monitor your heart rate manually, stop or slow down after a few minutes of exercising, and within three seconds, count the pulse at your neck, wrist, temple, or chest for six seconds. To take your pulse from your neck, wrist, or temple, place the tips of the index and middle fingers (not the thumb, which has a pulse of its own) over the artery and press lightly. When taking your pulse on your chest, place the heel of your right hand over the left side of your chest. At the same time, look at a second hand on a clock or watch and count the number of times you feel a pulse for six seconds.

When you have the number of beats for six seconds, multiply that number by ten. That number represents how many times your heart is beating per minute during that particular exercise. That number should be in your zone. If you're not in your zone, adjust your intensity level by either raising or lowering the intensity until you are in your zone. Take your pulse a number of times during exercise. With practice, you won't have to check your pulse as often—you'll know by how you're feeling how hard you're working. If during your workout you experience shortness of breath, are unable to talk comfortably during aerobic activity, or experience dizziness or a feeling of nausea, stop exercising immediately. Place a wet, cool towel on your head and lie down on your back with your feet level with your head.

It's also critical to know your heart rate zone before you begin exercising. It will save you time figuring out whether you need to adjust your intensity during your workout. Another popular means of measuring intensity during exercise is by "perceived exertion." Rather than use a formula, Borg's scale—the rate of perceived exertion (RPE)—was developed to allow exercisers to subjectively rate their feelings during exercise, taking into account personal fitness level, environmental conditions, and general fatigue levels. Currently, two RPE scales are widely used: the original, which rates exercise intensity on a scale of 6–20; and the revised scale of 0–10. This revised and simplified scale uses terminology that's easier to understand, thereby providing the tester with more valid information by which to further direct the test. Both scales account for the increase in heart rate during exercise.

The RPE scale is especially valuable because it provides exercisers of all fitness

Revised Scales for Ratings of Perceived Exertion (RPE):

0	Nothing at all
0.5	Very, very weak
1	Very weak
2	Weak
3	Moderate
4	Somewhat strong
5	Strong
6	
7	Very Strong
8	
9	
10	Very, very strong
—	Maximal

Taken from the American College of Sports Medicine's *Guidelines for Exercise Testing & Prescription,* 5th Edition, 1995

levels with easily understood guidelines regarding exercise intensity.

The best thing about the Borg scale is that it does not require any math or formulas. While exercising, simply ask yourself how you rate your exertion, from 0 to 10. If you feel that you are at a 3, then you can pick up your intensity. After rating your exertion, you can take your pulse. Your pulse should fall somewhere in the zone that you've chosen, according to your goals. I recommend this scale primarily for regular exercisers and healthy subjects. If you have special needs, including a heart condition, I recommend using a heart rate monitor to ensure your safety.

How to Raise Your Intensity

If your goal is to increase your fitness level, you will need to increase your intensity level. This can be achieved by increasing either the time (duration), the speed, the resistance, or a combination of any of these three elements in your exercise regimen. For instance, if you walk on a treadmill for twenty minutes at a zero level (without an incline) at a speed of 3 mph, and your heart rate measures 130 beats per minute, two weeks later, that same walk will only push your heart rate up to 120 beats per minute. If you don't increase your intensity, then you won't increase your fitness level. You won't burn as many calories as you did at 130 beats per minute, you will not become more cardiovascularly fit, and you will not improve how your body looks.

It's important to raise your intensity gradually, so that injury does not occur. If you're just beginning an exercise program, it's best to increase your intensity by increasing your time (duration). If you're moderately fit, I'd suggest increasing the resistance (walking on an incline, for example), coupled with increasing duration. And if you're fit, increase both your resistance and your speed. The more fit you become, the easier it will be to increase your intensity.

Increasing intensity is very demanding mentally as well as physically, but it's extremely important to keep increasing intensity until you have met your fitness and aesthetic goals. When you have reached the point of true fitness, you no longer need to increase your intensity. At this point, you only need to maintain your fitness level. That's the ultimate goal— getting your body to become fit enough to maintain your level of fitness.

Achieving Your Goals

No matter what your goals, there should be no difference in how you approach your fitness program: whether you want to exercise to improve your golf game or your overall health, to lose weight, to acquire bigger muscles, or simply to tone your body, you still must be organized and make the right choices before you begin. Often, what you set out to do falls short because you didn't do all your homework before you began exercising. For instance, let's say you enjoy playing golf in the spring and summer. You have a very hectic lifestyle and schedule, so you don't think you have time to exercise or to train properly for the upcoming golf season. Before you know it, spring has arrived and you suddenly decide to work out to "get in shape." You start working out three to four days a week, and because you're pressed for time (to start golfing in two weeks), you overdo it and injure yourself.

In reality, you should have been exercising two to three days a week year-round. If you suddenly can find the time to exercise when the golf season is upon you, why not before? The good news is that you have found something to motivate you to exercise; now you just need to maintain that motivation.

The point is this: no matter what your reason or motivation to exercise, you need to be honest with yourself about your expectations, based on the effort you're willing to put toward your fitness and aesthetic goals. As I often ask my clients, how successful would you be at your work or career if you only went to work occasionally, say, one day a week? As a golfer, you need to devote time and effort to exercise and fitness if you expect to hit the ball with more power and distance. If you only choose to exercise every once in a while, that's okay, but don't complain that you hate the way you're playing golf or how you look and feel because, quite simply, you haven't earned the right to do so!

The key question you need to ask yourself when assessing your goals and deciding what you want out of your fitness regimen is this: will I be able to do all, or at least most, of the exercises I'm currently performing on a consistent basis three to five days a week, week after week? Of course, you may need to make minor adjustments here and there along the way, but, as I have stressed throughout this chapter, your success in reaching your fitness goals has more to do with planning before you begin exercising than the actual act of exercising itself.

Let me help you define your goal—and improve your golf game—by categorizing the exercises for bodies that are evenly portioned, top-heavy, or bottom-heavy. Making your body a little more symmetrical and balanced throughout is essential for hitting the golf ball farther and playing better golf.

Match Your Workouts to Your Goals

Whether you need to improve your flexibility to follow through on your swing, increase your strength to hit the ball farther, lose weight for greater mobility, or improve your eye-hand coordination and timing, *Fit to a Tee* has exercises to address your specific golf goals.

The most difficult thing to figure out when exercising is the correct percentage of aerobic versus anaerobic exercise you need in order to achieve either your weight loss or toning goals. Aerobic exercises are primarily for weight loss, and anaerobic exercises are better suited for toning your body. That being said, it's imperative to know and follow certain principles so that your body changes in ways that enable it to function more efficiently, and your motivation remains high so that you continue to work out regularly. In the box on the next page are some guiding principles to help you determine how to maximize your exercise time to effectively reach your golf, fitness, and aesthetic goals.

Fitness Guidelines

Goals:

- If you are overweight and want to lose weight, you need to focus on exercises that are best suited for weight loss, such as stationary biking, walking, jogging, jumping rope, or any other aerobic-type exercise of your choice.

- If you have a slight frame and want to add weight to your body, you need to do more anaerobic-type exercises, such as chin-ups, dips, weightlifting, and any other form of strengthening exercises.

- The heavier you are, the lighter the weights and resistance you should use so that you don't build up more muscle under your fat.

- The lighter you are, the more weight and resistance you should use so that you add mass to your body.

- If you want to rid your midsection of extra flab, you need to perform both aerobic (to shed the outer layer of fat) and anaerobic exercises (to firm muscles).

- If you are top-heavy, use lighter weights and resistance for all exercises when working that region of your body.

- If you are bottom-heavy, use lighter weights and resistance for all exercises when working that region of your body.

- If you are evenly proportioned and not overweight, you can use moderate weights and resistance for both your upper and lower body.

- If you are evenly proportioned but overweight, you should use only light weights and resistance for both your upper and lower body.

Please note: as you lose more weight, you can increase the amount of weights and resistance for each exercise, but not until you have lost some weight and inches; otherwise, you will not decrease the overall size of your body.

Frequency:

- For weight loss, you need to perform aerobic exercise five days a week for at least thirty minutes.

- If your goal is to add weight to your body, you need to perform high-intensity anaerobic exercise three days a week for at least forty-five minutes.

- If your goal is just to tone your body and you are not overweight, you need to perform more anaerobic-type exercises three days a week for at least thirty minutes.

- If your goal is to both lose weight and tone a bit, you need to perform at least twenty minutes of aerobic and twenty minutes of anaerobic exercise four days a week.

Please note: if you are trying to lose weight, you can shave off a day or two of aerobic exercise if and only if you adjust your diet and reduce your weekly total caloric intake. If you are trying to gain weight, you must increase your total caloric intake.

Additional Guidelines

All of the principles spelled out in this chapter are based on medical science and the more than twenty years of practical experience I have gathered working with people from all walks of life. You cannot arbitrarily pick and choose your own guidelines based on your dietary and exercise preferences. If you want to lose weight but choose not to perform aerobic exercise five days week, or don't adjust your diet by drastically decreasing the amount of food you're ingesting, you might initially lose some weight, but you will not achieve your total weight loss goals. You must adapt these principles to your lifestyle. So save yourself a lot of time, headaches, and frustration, and do it correctly from the start.

If you need to increase your flexibility and/or range of motion, you should stretch every day for at least ten minutes—even on days when you are not exercising. On days when you are exercising, of course, you will already be stretching before your workout and may want to stretch a bit afterward, as well.

In summary, use common sense and be fair and honest with yourself as you attempt to reach your goals. If you are overweight and cannot work out one day because of a constraint, pay careful attention to your diet that day so as not to gain a pound or two. On the other hand, if you have been working out regularly and are a bit sore or fatigued, take a day off here or there and just keep yourself active on days when you are not exercising.

Maximizing Your Exercise Time

Now you know the five components of fitness (page 15). What elements must your fitness regimen contain to help you succeed in becoming fit? Various fitness and exercise experts encourage new exercisers to pick and choose exercises they will "like." We have become a society seeking to do the least amount of work necessary, yet we want instant gratification with great results. And we wonder why we look, feel, and function on only one cylinder and in first gear year-round. It's not really a matter of "liking" an exercise. If it is safe, efficient, and effective, and it will improve your golf game and make you look and feel better, believe me, you'll start to like it. If we don't follow the steps necessary to improve our overall fitness, we really won't give ourselves a chance to realize the rewards that come from proper fitness. If you alter the sequence and vary the amounts and types of exercises necessary to succeed, you will not become fit. I cannot emphasize this enough, so please heed my advice and follow all the instructions that follow to ensure that you will feel and look your best all year round!

The Four Phases of Exercise

There are four phases of exercise—warm-up, stretch, workload, and cool-down—and you must perform your exercise routine in this exact order every time you work out to maximize benefits and avoid injury. Each phase is equally important and allows you to progress within the framework of your exercise routines. I guarantee that you will become more fit and thus more motivated to sustain consistency. So, as you can see, it's vital to understand and follow these four phases, even if you don't like them.

I'm always amazed to discover that only a handful of current exercisers start their workout with a proper warm-up! I'm even more astonished when people who have worked with personal trainers don't know the difference between warming up and stretching, or they have no working knowledge of when or how to stretch properly.

Educate yourself on the exercises best suited for you, be consistent, and the rest will take care of itself. This book is intended to show that we all can improve our current level of fitness, and that fitness improves your golf game and all other aspects of your day-to-day life. If you are currently exercising and it has not carried over to hitting the golf ball farther and your body is not changing for the better, it must be because of a problem that has not yet been identified or corrected. But don't despair: by the end of this book you will be able to figure out how you need to change your fitness regimen in order to succeed.

The Warm-Up

Warming up is the first phase of your workout. Warming up is not stretching, and stretching is not warming up. There are many people who confuse the two.

Warning: don't stretch until you've warmed up.

The warm-up accomplishes several things: it raises your heart rate from its resting state gradually and safely in order to prepare your heart for more demanding activity; it provides a smooth transition from the resting state to the higher level of energy expenditure in the main part of your workout, called the workload; it prepares the body physiologically and psychologically for physical performance, and also lessens the possibility of injury; it raises both the general body temperature and the deep muscle temperature, and stretches collagen tissues, which permits greater flexibility; and it increases your physical working capacity during your workout.

Do you have any idea of the torque to your body when you swing a golf club? If you did, you would definitely warm up and stretch before each round. The back and torso area absorb the most shock, and when you put too many demands on your system, the body cannot adapt to the shock unless it's properly lubricated.

Failing to warm up properly is especially detrimental to those who are just beginning an exercise program or taking up the game of golf. In fact, most heart attacks that occur during exercise or strenuous activities, such as shoveling snow or mowing the lawn, could have been prevented if the person had warmed up first. Here's why: the warm-up gradually raises your heart rate from its resting state to a higher level. Certain movements raise your heart rate quickly. If your heart rate rises too quickly, the stress on the heart becomes compounded, and for those whose hearts are not well conditioned, this could bring on a heart attack.

Proper Ways to Warm Up

General warm-up procedures should consist of jogging, walking, easy running, stationary biking, working on an elliptical machine or a cross-trainer, swimming, rowing, or other light aerobic activity. The intensity of the warm-up should match your current level of fitness. The more fit you are, the more aggressive you can be in your warm-up. The reason is simple: your heart is in better shape and as your fitness increases, your body must meet new challenges to maintain that fitness level.

Warning: do not lift weights as a way to warm up; it raises your heart rate too quickly. Only warm up by performing aerobic activity.

Your time frame for warming up will vary anywhere from five to fifteen minutes. The more fit you are, the shorter the time you need. It should be of sufficient duration and intensity so that your body feels loose and you start to break a steady sweat, without developing marked fatigue. The colder the weather, the longer you'll need to warm up

Another important factor to consider is the type of exercise or activity in which you'll be engaging. Try to warm up in a way that corresponds to your fitness regimen. For instance, if you choose to use jogging/running as your main aerobic exercise, warm

up by jogging, perhaps on a treadmill, if one is available, for ten minutes or so. Why? Because the same muscle groups will be more taxed and utilized later on during your workout.

Warning: you need to warm up even before engaging in leisure activities like golf. Any sport or activity that raises the heart rate considerably; utilizes fast movements; or requires your body to use a wide range of motion requires a warm-up. If you don't regularly engage in a particular sport or activity, I recommend warming up with a stationary bike. It's small, relatively inexpensive, and you can adjust the tension (resistance) according to your fitness level readily and easily. In addition, you only utilize 50 to 60 percent of your body weight while biking as opposed to walking on a treadmill, which requires you to move your entire body. This is especially important if you have a heart condition because your heart rate will not rise as quickly if the tension on the bike is low.

Now that you've completed your warm-up, you're ready for the second phase of your workout: stretching.

Stretching

Try to make sure that no more than five minutes elapses between completing your warm-up and stretching. The key to increasing your flexibility is warming up first and then stretching the major muscle groups in a sequential manner. So you need to perform a group of stretches in a precise order to increase your flexibility and prepare your body for the workload and stress that

Be sure to warm up and stretch before working out

you'll be putting on your muscles (see chapter 6 on how to stretch properly).

There are many reasons for stretching and they're all equally important. If your goal is to become stronger, you must stretch. If you want to get rid of your saddlebags, you'd better stretch. If you want to exercise injury-free, you need to stretch. And if you want to hit the golf ball farther and with more power and a greater range of motion, you must stretch! If you don't stretch, you will never achieve your fitness goals. Stretching also promotes circulation, and makes you feel good.

Stretching does not require a lot of time—only about three to five minutes, depending on your current level of flexibility. For some, flexibility comes easily; for others, it is the most uncomfortable part of working out. As you age, you need to spend a little more time stretching. And if you lack flexibility, you need to spend a few more minutes stretching as well. The rule is this: the more flexible you are, the less you need to stretch. If you have tight hamstrings but flexible quadriceps, spend a little more time stretching your hamstrings. Stretching increases your range of motion, which, in turn, will allow your muscles to grow faster and respond faster. Want to send every golf shot farther? You can add at least twenty yards to your distance or fifteen to thirty miles per hour to your swing speed simply by increasing your range of motion. You can take all the golf lessons in the world, but if you have poor flexibility, it will be hard to improve your distance and swing speed. And

that doesn't apply to golf alone. You can enhance your performance in any sport by modestly improving your flexibility.

Consider two people of the same age with the same body type, height, weight, and genetic makeup. If one stretched and the other did not, the one who stretched would have better body tone, would be more fit, and would also hit the golf ball much farther. I know this is true, not just because every medical journal has stated it, but because of the many frustrated and unhappy regular exercisers I have seen and advised, as well as those with whom I've played golf. There they are, sweating and sweating and thinking and hoping that one day their body will change for the better, but it never does. Although genetics does play a role in flexibility, you can greatly increase your flexibility if you learn the correct stretching techniques. I know plenty of athletes who are tremendously strong but are constantly pulling muscles, especially their hamstrings (located on the back of the leg). This is usually due to overtraining and lack of flexibility, or a lack of proper training coupled with poor flexibility.

Certain types of exercise can either increase or decrease your flexibility, depending on your form, the number of times the exercise is repeated, the range of motion used, and many other factors. For example, jogging and running tend to tighten your hamstrings; biking tightens the quadriceps (the front of your thighs); and weightlifting, especially powerlifting, can

> **Stretching reduces the chance of injury, promotes circulation, and feels good**

tighten the entire body, especially the shoulder and back region.

Please be aware that stretching will not prevent all injuries, but if you stretch, the likelihood of injury is much less than if you did not stretch. Good flexibility increases your ability to avoid injury; since it permits a greater range of movement within your joints, the ligaments and other collagenous tissues are not as easily strained or torn. It also allows for greater freedom of movement in all directions. Conversely, hyperflexibility must be avoided, because loose-jointed individuals are more prone to dislocations and other injuries. Extremes in flexibility are of little value and can result in weakness of the joint at certain angles. Flexibility for golf, in particular, is quite specific to the joint and its surrounding complementary tissues. This varies, however, from one person to the next.

The proper way to stretch is a relaxed, sustained stretch called static stretching. The wrong way is to bounce up and down (ballistic), or to stretch until you feel pain, which can do more harm than good. Only world-class athletes participating in certain sports practice ballistic stretching.

When you stretch, hold the stretch for thirty to sixty seconds. Do this with every stretch. Hold a static stretch so that the specific joint is immobilized in a position that places the desired muscles and connective tissues at their greatest possible length. There is little risk of injury if you perform static stretching.

Stretch until you feel a mild tension, and relax as you hold the stretch. The feeling of tension should subside slightly as you hold the stretch. If it does not, ease off a bit and find a degree of tension that is comfortable. If you can, stretch slightly farther and

continue to hold the position. Again, the tension should lessen; if not, ease off slightly. While stretching, breathe normally. Exhale as you bend into the stretch and continue breathing as you hold your stretch. Do not hold your breath while stretching, and remember to relax your facial muscles. If a stretch position prohibits you from breathing normally, ease up on the stretch in order to breathe more easily. In the beginning, silently count the seconds for each stretch. As you gain experience, you will be able to hold the stretch without counting, but, rather, based on how it feels. At the end of this chapter, you'll find an easy sequence of stretches to follow.

Please note that if you are very inflexible, I recommend stretching for a few minutes at the end of your workout, after you have cooled down. But be careful how much you stretch and how vigorously you stretch, especially if you worked out hard and taxed a particular region of your body during your workout, because you can also pull a muscle while stretching. For example, if you have tight hamstrings (which most people do) and you just jogged five miles and worked your legs earlier, perform a light hamstring stretch because these muscles are fatigued and will not be able to absorb much more shock. You can, however, aggressively stretch your core section or upper body that day. By contrast, when you work more of your upper body on a different workout day, you can aggressively stretch your hamstrings. If you are very inflexible (yes, guys, this is specifically addressed at you), I would recommend taking a yoga class. Yoga by itself, though, is not sufficient to make you fit, so you still need to do other exercises in order to become completely fit.

You are now ready for the third phase of your workout, called the workload.

The Workload

Often confused with the workout, the workload portion of your fitness routine must be well organized and orchestrated before you start exercising. Your workload segment is when you exercise at the highest intensity; by warming up and stretching, you've gotten your body prepared for this phase. In fact, you cannot effectively train at a high intensity unless you have warmed up and stretched. That is one of the main purposes of warming up and stretching. But your workload is the "nucleus" of your fitness regimen. If you have allotted an hour and fifteen minutes for your workout (ten minutes for warm-up, five minutes for stretching), you now have sixty minutes to fill: fifty-five to fifty-eight minutes for the workload and two to three minutes for cooling down. Those fifty-eight minutes or so need to be divided based on your goals (lose weight, tone, get in shape for golf), your body type (which will dictate the variety of exercises you should be performing), your orthopedic and medical background (dictating which exercises you shouldn't be performing), and your present level of fitness (determining the amount of intensity—low, moderate, or high).

That's why it's imperative to know how to perform all your exercises properly before you start exercising. You should transition smoothly into your workload right after you've stretched. Your combination of exercises needs to be choreographed like a waltz or ballet, with total focus. You may speak to others while you're warming up or stretching, but during your workload, you need to be completely immersed and selfishly block out any outside distractions.

If you work out at a gym or health club, the next time you're there notice all the people talking, laughing, and watching others when they're supposed to be engrossed in their own workout. Working out at a health club today has become a social event. I find it harder to concentrate on exercising in a health club than when I work out at a small gym or even at home. In my experience, the people who work out at home are more fit, better educated about fitness, more focused, and more consistent in their exercise routine than those who work out at a health club. People who exercise at home tend to integrate their workout into their lifestyle better than other exercisers.

Your average time for your workload, unless you're training for a competitive sport (in which case the time will differ depending on the sport), will be anywhere from forty-five to sixty minutes. You have a number of options as to how you're going to split up that time. Let's say you've got fifty minutes for your workload phase, you're moderately fit, and your goal is to lose weight (approximately forty pounds). Well, you already know the correct percentage of aerobic versus anaerobic exercise (see chapter 3), so most of your workload will consist of moderately intense aerobic work with some anaerobic exercises blended in. How do you know what to do and when to do it?

The rule of thumb is this: perform the exercises that you dislike the most and get them out of the way first. I suggest that you do twenty to thirty minutes of aerobic work and intersperse aerobics between segments of short periods of abdominal exercises and some upper body exercises. If you don't enjoy stomach work, do it right after your first stint of cardio work, because if you wait until the end of your workload to perform the exercises that you loathe, most likely you'll never do them.

The Importance of Intensity

Learning how and when to increase the intensity during the workload phase of your workout takes some practice. Once you've "mastered" one exercise, taking it to the next level requires mental toughness. For instance, if you're jumping rope for two minutes and you're out of breath, instead of stopping and giving up, get on a stationary bike or walk around for a minute or two, allowing your heart rate to come down a bit, then go right back to that jump rope for another minute or so in order to intensify your cardiovascular conditioning. You must increase your intensity in order to raise your fitness level. To do this safely, you must be in tune with your body and know how to perform each exercise properly. Remember that four months from now your workouts will be far different from what they are the first few times.

As you progress with your exercise program, you need to up your intensity, whether you take exercise classes, lift weights, work out on weight machines, run, swim, row, or practice any other form of exercise. How do you know when you've reached the optimum intensity level? You need to keep increasing intensity until you've met the following criteria: your fitness program is well balanced, meaning you have good flexibility, muscle strength, muscle endurance, cardiovascular efficiency, and a good body ratio of lean body mass to fat; you can participate in a sport you enjoy, like golf, at a level that completely satisfies you; you're pleased with your weight and body fat percentage; you've met all your health goals, including proper blood pressure, cholesterol level, and resting heart rate; you fit comfortably in your clothes; you look and feel great!

Increasing the intensity of your exercise regimen is a skill that can be learned with patience and practice. I emphasize patience because too often people who exercise, especially those who are just starting out, want to be fit in a week or so. Others want to lose fifteen pounds in two weeks. My point is that when you try to be overly aggressive with your fitness regimen, you're bound to injure yourself. Remember, if you injure yourself while exercising, you cannot be consistent, and if you're not consistent, you'll never reach your goals. Most importantly, if you're hurt, you cannot play golf, so you'll be hurt and miserable at the same time.

Knowing precisely what to do during your workload becomes more important as you boost your fitness level. Keeping yourself on track is also a more efficient way to exercise, because most people must work out within the time parameters they've laid out and stick to them. One mistake people often make as they become more fit is to add new exercises to their regimen that involve new pieces of fitness equipment. But while they're adding new exercises, they aren't eliminating others, and if you don't do that, you'll be exercising for hours on end. You need to learn to increase your intensity using the same fitness equipment, as well as when to add new exercises and when to drop those that are no longer as effective as they once were. As you become more fit and lean, if you have not reached all your goals, then you have to keep increasing the intensity until you reach the maintenance stage.

Contrary to popular belief, you do not need to dramatically alter your routine and change the exercises you're performing in order to keep increasing your intensity.

When you think you've hit a plateau, don't completely change your exercise regimen. Have you noticed that professional athletes never seem to plateau? That's because they keep increasing the intensity of the fitness routines they are doing. Perhaps you have plateaued because you aren't exercising often enough, or maybe you're exercising incorrectly based on your goals, or—as in

Tips on the Workload

Here are some simple, easy-to-understand guidelines for increasing your exercise intensity: if you're less to moderately fit, increase your time for all aerobic activities and the number of the repetitions for all anaerobic exercises; if you're more fit, increase the resistance (make sure that it matches your aesthetic goals) for all aerobic activities and add more weight for all anaerobic exercises, when applicable. The important things to remember about your workload are the following:

- To raise your fitness level and change your body, you need to increase your intensity.

- As you become more fit, keep increasing your intensity in some way in order to burn sufficient fat and calories.

- If you're relatively unfit, it's safer to increase your intensity by extending the time you exercise (duration) and the number of repetitions—rather than the resistance. This will help prevent serious injury.

- Once you've mastered an exercise (with proper form and number of repetitions), either switch to a new exercise or make the exercise more intense.

- When and if you choose to lift moderate to heavy weights, be careful to avoid quick, jerky movements.

- If you're sore from performing a certain exercise, ease up and rest the part of your body that feels tender until the soreness subsides.

- To ensure maximum results, make sure that before you start your workload phase you fully understand the purpose and proper form of any exercises you will be performing.

- On days that you need to shorten your workout time (duration), make sure that you still warm up and stretch before the workload phase of your fitness regimen, and that you cool down afterward.

most cases I've encountered—maybe you're not exercising with enough intensity, combined with the wrong exercises.

Too often, what you read, hear, or see dictates what you do when it comes to exercise. Just as you would be careful to choose the proper golf pro or instructor to help you with your golf swing, you should seek out advice on exercise and fitness carefully.

The Cool-Down

The cool-down is the shortest phase of your workout. Typically, it lasts between three and five minutes, depending on the intensity of your workout. The cool-down has many functions and is often overlooked or performed improperly. Remember, it only takes a couple of minutes to complete, but the repercussions are severe if you skip it.

Another way of understanding the cool-down process is this: when you start your workout by warming up, your heart rate gradually rises. Then during your workout it continues to rise considerably, and remains high for an extended period of time. In order to bring your heart rate back down toward your pre-exercise level, you need to keep moving your body but at a gradually decreasing intensity. Viewed another way, the cool-down is the exact opposite of the warm-up, yet not as long or intense.

How long you should cool down is dictated by how long and how intense your

workout has been. Anywhere from three to five minutes should be sufficient, depending on the intensity of the workload phase. If you feel you need more time, then take a few extra minutes. Your breathing should return to normal and your pulse should return to under one hundred beats per minute within a few minutes of finishing your workload phase. By properly and sufficiently cooling down, you greatly reduce your chance of experiencing cardiac complications, especially if you have any type of heart problem. It's the sudden cessation of exercise that you're trying to avoid with the cool-down.

An effective way to cool down is to engage in mild aerobic-type exercises—stationary biking (with little or no tension), walking (with no elevation or hills), slow jogging, leisurely swimming, rowing (with no resistance), and getting on a cross-trainer or an elliptical machine with no incline are the best and safest options. Do not cool down by performing any anaerobic exercises; these will raise your heart rate rather than lower it. Don't ever skip the cool-down phase, even if you're pressed for time. You need to give your body time to readjust from your workload.

You're just about ready now to learn how to improve your fitness, thus allowing you to hit the golf ball farther, more accurately, and with more power. The next chapter will help you overcome any excuses or constraints that may prevent you from performing your workouts consistently.

Motivation: Committing to Exercise

You are now aware of what you need to know to succeed with proper and regular exercise. But you need to promise yourself that you are in this for the long haul—for the rest of your life, not just for a week or a few months. From time to time, you will have ups and downs with your fitness program, just as you might have hot and cold streaks with your golf game. But, with perseverance, you will improve in every area of fitness and exercise if you practice consistently. It is a process with a learning curve, and as time goes by, you will become better and better every time you exercise. To achieve your fitness goals, there are three key elements: you must have a solid plan, you must see positive results within thirty days, and your exercise plan must be simple yet effective—one that you can keep fine-tuning over time.

For this process to work, you first need to have a complete understanding of how exercise relates to your golf game and what you want out of your fitness program. When

it comes to exercise, there is a direct correlation between education and motivation. You need to educate yourself about the best way for you to exercise based on your lifestyle, medical and orthopedic background, present level of fitness, and most important, your goals. These four factors are crucial in building and sustaining your motivation. That motivation will carry over to your golf game, because the fitter you become, the farther you will hit the golf ball and the better your golf game will be.

Making a strong commitment to regular exercise does not happen overnight. True, some of us have a greater ability to motivate ourselves to work out than others, but all of us are capable of building the habit of fitness into our daily life. Too many times, we find ourselves negotiating whether to exercise. Time constraints, fatigue, travel, and the like soon become excuses. Developing the commitment to exercise is a learned trait, a trait that only becomes a habit in phases and stages. Take the steps you need to form this important habit.

You must be savvy when it comes to fitness because it can be a very frustrating experience. Hard work and consistency still do not guarantee that you will become fit or build a good body. It's similar to the guy or gal who goes to the range and spends countless hours hitting balls but is not practicing correctly. This is why it is so important to educate yourself and define your goals before you start your exercise regimen.

Another tip to help you build your commitment to exercise is to take a step backward and prioritize what's important in your life. In addition to becoming a better golfer and hitting the golf ball farther and with more power, slotting fitness into your life will help you improve your health, gain more energy, reduce stress, increase your longevity, enhance your relationships, combat depression and, best of all, increase your self-confidence.

The Centers for Disease Control surveyed a large group of people who were not exercising and found that 70 percent of them said that the number-one reason they did not engage in a regular fitness regimen was that they did not know how to fit it into their lifestyle. Unfortunately, we possess limited knowledge about how to make exercise part of our daily lives. Whatever reason you have for not exercising, it all boils down to lack of motivation. But that's only one hurdle. If

you're fortunate enough to possess the motivation to exercise, you still need to retrain your mind and body, and learn how to motivate yourself to exercise properly.

Here's one of the biggest misconceptions about lifestyle and fitness: most people think that in order to start or maintain an exercise regimen, they must change their current lifestyle and exercise a few hours every day to reach their goals. Your lifestyle, as crazy and busy as it is, should not interfere with maintaining your fitness regimen. However, it can get in the way of your motivation to make the time for exercise. For example, say you really are not that motivated to exercise in the first place and you have a very hectic day-to-day schedule, plus you want to practice and play golf a certain number of times a week or month. The odds are against you succeeding in your pursuit of regular exercise. To increase those odds, you are going to have to learn how to work out despite your busy schedule, because your lifestyle is not going to get any less hectic.

I can't tell you how many times over the years people have said to me, "Edward, let me call you in a couple of weeks when things calm down for me." You may have used this excuse yourself. I always counter with, "What's going to change in a couple of weeks?" In a few weeks you're going to tell me the same thing. In my many years of dealing with time management, I have found that people are indeed busy, but it's not their busyness that prevents them from exercising regularly. Most of them are

> **Committing to exercise is a learned trait**

poorly organized and have limited time-management skills, not just when it comes to fitness, but in all facets of their lives. They are always rushing, never meeting deadlines, and, of course, not exercising. That's the symptom, not the cause. The only way to exercise consistently is to change the way you manage your day-to-day activities—that's the true cause of your failure to exercise regularly.

Whether you realize it or not, you use your lifestyle as an excuse for not exercising. It's an easy out. Until now, fitness was never important enough for you to find a solution to your dilemma. Or maybe you've never experienced the benefits of a consistent exercise regimen. People constantly look—sometimes not even consciously—for excuses not to exercise. Whether your excuse is real or perceived, it doesn't matter, because it is still getting in the way of maintaining your fitness regimen.

How many times have you put off doing a chore or something important? You know that the more you procrastinate, the worse it gets because now you are not putting your full energy toward all the other things that need attention. After a while, you find yourself always rushing around, disorganized, and never quite finding the time to take care of all your day-to-day responsibilities—you're always playing catch-up. Well, the same thing happens when you keep putting off your responsibility to exercise. You either try to make it up on weekends or never address your fitness needs at all. By doing so, you never realize how much better you can look and feel with proper and regular exercise.

This chapter examines the most common excuses used to stall your efforts

toward fitness and how you can combat them. Some of you may have more than one constraint on your time or your energy. Sometimes certain incidents or stressors in life prompt you to create "layers" of excuses that prevent you from working out consistently. In this chapter, you will finally learn how to stop focusing on the symptom and start treating the cause of your inconsistent approach to exercise.

The first step in developing a sound fitness regimen is creating a clear path for regular and proper fitness, despite any obstacles in your life. Although you may be somewhat motivated to exercise, if you haven't eliminated the barriers to being consistent in your workout regimen, you will never succeed in meeting your goal of increasing your distance hitting the golf ball.

You may think after reading the excuses for not exercising, spelled out on the following pages, that your reason is not included, but believe me, it's in there, either in whole or in part. As you read, identify which obstacles you need to overcome and then tackle them. Never lose confidence, and never think to yourself, "My golf game will never really be that great," or "My body will never change—I'm stuck with it this way for the rest of my life."

We all can improve our fitness level and see not only a positive change in our overall golf game but also a positive change in our body. Your excuse for not exercising properly and consistently is hidden in one of these ten constraints. Try to find your excuse and apply the solutions I'm offering.

I Have a Hectic Lifestyle.
I'm a family man with a high-stress job. I drive to work one hour each way, and have three

children and my wife to tend to when I get home in the evening. I've tried to balance my career and family in relation to my workouts. With my hectic lifestyle, I'm not sure I can exercise during the workweek—I don't have enough time. On weekends I'm able to exercise, but my golf dates with my buddies often take precedence. How am I ever going to be able to work out during the week with my current schedule? I'm trying to lose about twenty pounds, and on weekends I drop about two pounds, but during the week I seem to gain it back. I'm very frustrated.

Solution

Your predicament is the number-one reason why people don't exercise—a hectic lifestyle. Whether you're a commuter, a busy homemaker, travel frequently, work long hours or entertain, fitting exercise into your lifestyle seems impossible, but with time, it will become a learned trait. The key here is organization. You need to sit down with your spouse and come up with a schedule that allows you time—either when you come home or before leaving for work—that is yours alone. You have many options here, but before I give you the steps to solve your problem, you need to recognize that educating yourself about exercise should be your top priority. You should have three workouts from which to choose: a long workout (one hour), for when time allows; a thirty-minute routine; and a weekend workout that can be performed in and around your golf and other family obligations. The key is to understand how to exercise efficiently within your allotted time frame. Be careful here, because when you're up against a time constraint and you aren't sure what to do, by the time you figure out which exercises

to perform, your allotted time will have passed. Further, if you only have a limited time for fitness, you're more apt to exercise for that thirty minutes if you know in advance what to do. If you don't know how to exercise with only thirty minutes, that will become yet another excuse.

The following steps will help you get organized. Step 1: Decide where and when you will be working out. Will it be at home, or at a health club near home or work? Choose the place that will be most convenient—and keep you coming back. You might even choose more than one location—it doesn't matter, as long as you're consistent about it. Step 2: Educate yourself about the type of exercise regimen that you'll be able to perform on a regular basis, a routine that you can maintain given your lifestyle parameters. Step 3: Even if you only have thirty minutes and you're disappointed that you can't get your one-hour routine in, do the thirty-minute routine anyway. You might have to perform it more frequently to achieve your weight loss goals, but you're still establishing the habit of exercising.

Am I Exercising Wrong?

I'm a businesswoman in advertising and I'm always giving presentations, so how I look and feel is paramount to my profession. I know you won't believe this, but since I've been lifting weights and exercising, I've actually gained mass and size, and my legs, butt, hips, and arms look like a football player's. A number of women in my golfing group have commented that I look like I've gained weight, but I haven't gained a pound! It's not as if I'm overeating, either—I watch my diet carefully every day. I keep hoping that my body will take a turn for the better, but it hasn't. I no longer feel as motivated to work out as I did when I started.

Solution

This is a classic case of not exercising properly for your body type. Many thousands of women and men experience this dilemma. The good news is that, despite your current shape, you can change it for the better if you change your workout regimen. Some people have a tendency to bulk up faster than others in certain areas of their body. Their genetic and biological makeup allows muscle mass to build faster than they can lose fat, if their fitness regimen is incorrect. The best advice I can give you is to relax, don't worry about what others are thinking, and stay focused on the benefits of fitness. And you need to revamp your workout so that you will start to see the fruits of your hard labor—otherwise you'll never lose that bulk.

The most difficult thing for many of us is accepting the need for change. When people get stuck in their fitness regimen, it is not easy for them to get out. You know one thing for sure—whatever you're doing now isn't working, plain and simple. You also know that in order to slim down more, you need to figure out how to change your current routine. Regardless of your gender, if you're lifting weights and you don't want to add bulk, high repetition combined with light weights is the correct formula for you. After a few weeks, your body will start changing for the better. The best way for me to motivate you to continue exercising is to assure you that proper exercise will help you improve the way you look. If you were willing to exercise incorrectly for years without seeing the desired changes in your body, then you certainly should be motivated to work out properly once you start seeing those changes. As your body starts responding in a more positive way, you'll be able to wear those sleeveless shirts proudly and your girlfriends will stop snickering!

I'm Too Tired to Exercise.

By the end of the day, I'm exhausted, and believe me, the last thing I think of doing is exercise. My work is very mentally demanding and stressful. Each morning I wake up tired, and it takes me a while to get my motor running in the morning. I just don't have the energy and motivation to work out. In fact, the very thought of doing any kind of physical exercise is exhausting. All I want to do is have a drink and watch television when I get home.

Solution

The primary reason you're so tired is that you're not moving enough. Unless you're a construction worker who moves around all day, you probably have no reason for being fatigued after work. Although your brain is being "exercised" on a regular basis, your body is sleeping. I know that you're tired, but unless you're tired from lack of sleep or from too much exercise, you should be exercising. The key here is to separate mental fatigue from physical sluggishness. This is a skill. Exercise will wake you up and allow you to sleep better, and you'll wake up with more zip. However, taking that first step is the most difficult. Once you get on that bike or treadmill, you'll get hooked. Since you like sitting and watching television, I suggest that you purchase a recumbent stationary bike; that way you can watch TV while you're exercising. Once you've biked about twenty minutes and you start to sweat, you'll gain energy—now you're ready psychologically and physiologically to continue with additional exercises. After finishing your biking, you'll feel revived. That feeling of being energized will help motivate you the next time you come home feeling tired. So the next time you think you're too tired to work out, think about the last time you were tired and you worked out anyway, and how wonderful you felt afterwards.

The increased energy level and general feeling of well-being that you experience each time you work out will keep you coming back for more. You'll see that fitness sometimes comes in phases and stages. It's important to get started, and in time, you'll move on to the next phase and add some exercises. Before you know it, you're doing things you thought you couldn't do. Remember, with fitness, what we want to do and should do, and what we actually end up doing, often do not match up. But as long as you're making positive strides toward incorporating a sound and regular fitness regimen into your lifestyle, you're on your way!

My Body Never Really Changed When I Did "Exercise."

I started exercising by walking and was able to keep it up for a couple of months, but I stopped because I didn't lose an ounce and didn't see any results. And, quite honestly, I didn't feel that much better than I did when I wasn't exercising.

Solution

Consider yourself lucky. Thousands have written and come to see me who've been exercising for five or ten years without any results! I don't blame you for becoming discouraged and quitting. Your lack of results could come from a combination of things: you might not be working out frequently enough, you could be exercising without enough intensity, or you have not reduced your daily caloric intake. But the main reason you don't feel better and have not seen the desired results is that walking, jogging, and the like do not equal fitness. Walking can be a part of your fitness regimen, but, by itself, it is not exercise. Walking will definitely improve your aerobic capacity for golf, but it falls far short of helping you lose weight and become fit and toned throughout your entire body. There could be at least ten additional reasons why people who share your dilemma have not reached their goals—there are many other factors that determine successful weight loss.

Let's say that you choose to do nothing but walk to lose weight. You still need to walk with enough intensity to match your current level of fitness, and you have to make sure that you are not eating more calories. For instance, if you start out by walking two miles a day in forty minutes, after a few weeks you need to increase your pace and walk those same two miles in less time. Your other option is to increase the distance you're walking, but the downside to this option is that now you need to increase the time you spend exercising, and that may not fit into your lifestyle. If you have an orthopedic constraint that prevents you from walking faster without putting undue stress on your joints, walking is not the most effective exercise for you to lose weight. You will need to switch to, perhaps, a stationary bike, which will allow you to peddle with higher intensity and burn more calories without stressing your joints.

Sometimes what we enjoy doing for exercise isn't what we need to do to reach our goals. Unless you accept this fact, you will never dramatically change the way you look and feel. That's why the best way to become—and stay—motivated is to learn more about what is best for your particular fitness goals. You'll find ways to reach your goals outlined in detail throughout this book.

I'm Looking for a Shortcut.

I just purchased my fourth piece of weight-lifting and toning fitness equipment from an infomercial. For the past four months, I've been following the directions exactly as prescribed, using the machine every other day for about twelve minutes, just as it says to on TV. How come I haven't lost weight and don't have the body I want?

Solution

Buying and using fitness equipment is no guarantee that you will improve your body. Nor is purchasing the fanciest, newest driver going to guarantee that you will hit the golf ball farther and with more accuracy. No one piece of fitness equipment by itself can make you fit. First off, stop taking shortcuts. Twelve minutes a couple of days a week? Not only do you need to spend more time with that particular gadget, but you also need to stretch and perform aerobic exercise for at least thirty minutes when you exercise. Proper fitness is not about owning a piece of exercise equipment, and unless you come to terms with that, you will continue to fail in your endeavors. Second, whether you purchase a piece of fitness equipment from TV or from a fitness store,

make sure you buy the best quality and that you will use it. Do not buy the cheapest piece of fitness equipment, because in the end you're not really saving money.

In addition, you must maintain an excellent diet. If weight loss is your goal, you are going to have to change your mindset about fitness, exercise, and nutrition. To lose weight, you must eat healthy foods and decrease your overall caloric intake. Even if you work out on all of your weight machines, you'll never lose weight and mass. How do we know this? Two ways: it would have worked already, and, scientifically speaking, in order to lose weight, aerobic—not anaerobic—exercise is what you need. This is a common dilemma, and although any form of proper weightlifting will build more muscle, it cannot convert your fat to muscle. Aerobic exercise will help you lose weight and mass. So, depending on how much weight you need to lose, you need the right formula of aerobic versus anaerobic exercise to reach your goals. You also need a caloric deficit to lose weight, so be conscious of your daily intake of food. Sometimes we eat more when we start an exercise program because we think we're already compensating for the extra calories by working out.

Instead of striving for a "perfect" body, focus your energies on pushing yourself to exercise with greater intensity within a more complete fitness program and eat sensibly. In time, you'll start looking "buff."

I Don't Enjoy Formal Exercise.

I really don't like exercising, but I do enjoy playing sports, especially skiing, tennis, and golf. I engage in these activities at least two days a week, so I get plenty of exercise.

Solution

There is a big misconception that golf, tennis, skiing, and other sports are synonymous with fitness. I'm not advising you to stop doing the things you enjoy, especially since one of the main functions of fitness is to be more active. But each time you exercise, your regimen must incorporate and promote the five components of fitness: flexibility, muscle endurance, muscle strength, cardiovascular conditioning, and body ratio (percent of lean muscle mass to fat). Tennis, skiing, and, yes, even golf at its most intense, aren't fitness regimens—they're sports and activities. And although you are very active, you'll never get fit simply by doing them. You cannot get fit just by being more active; you can be more active, however, by becoming more fit.

One of the best ways to motivate yourself to engage in regular exercise is to exercise or "train" specifically to enhance your sports performance. By doing sports-specific training, you will reduce your chances of injury, play at a much higher level, enjoy the sports for the sake of the sports themselves rather than relying on them as a form of exercise, gain confidence to try other activities that are a little more physically demanding, and be able to play your sports for many years to come, thus increasing your longevity.

Here's what you should do: two to three days a week, either before or right after you play your sport, do about thirty minutes of exercise that includes some aerobic work, stretching, and some strengthening exercises. Since you are already in your sports "mode," it's easier to keep you moving. As your performance in your sports and activities improves, you will be motivated to follow your exercise regimen with more regularity. Eventually, you will want to work out more often, separately from your sports.

It's Too Late for Me to Start.

I'm scared to start an exercise program. I'm forty pounds overweight, fifty-five years old, have a bad back, achy knees, and arthritis. I want to play golf more often, but I feel terrible after each round of golf and it takes me a few days to recover. Besides, what good will it do me now to get fit at this point in my life? I'll never be able to get in shape.

Solution

Being obese, overweight, or having medical concerns or orthopedic constraints are not acceptable excuses not to be exercising. In fact, these are important reasons to start a fitness regimen. One of the great things about proper exercise is that after you've been working out for a period of time, your body acts as if you've been working out your whole life. You're never too old to exercise, and if you wish to be old one day, I strongly suggest that you start exercising now. Too often, people are either misinformed or lack confidence in themselves. The key here is to start slowly and ease into a formal routine. Riding a recumbent stationary bike (one that you lean back in as opposed to sitting upright), for ten to twenty minutes at a low resistance, then stretching for a couple of minutes is a good start. (That's a gentle warm-up followed by stretching.) Once you build up some cardiovascular conditioning, then you can start to add a few other exercises. Don't compare yourself to anyone else. Concentrate on your goals and surround yourself with upbeat people who can help support you in your fitness pursuits.

Developing new relationships with people who are active and energetic will soon rub off on you in a positive way! I also suggest that you contact your local hospital's rehabilitation center and ask for an exercise specialist to work with you initially. As you better condition yourself, take some weight off, and strengthen your body, you will feel less torque after each round of golf, which will further motivate you.

I Always Get Injured When I Exercise.

Every time I gear myself up for exercising, I injure myself. Sometimes it's my back, or my knees become achy or I pull a muscle. Although I enjoy working out, my motivation is waning. By the time I recover from my injuries, I'm out of shape again. And it's really affecting my golf game; sometimes I can't play because it hurts to swing. I'm not getting any stronger with my current exercise regimen, which includes mostly weightlifting. I keep seesawing back and forth with my fitness level and now I'm afraid to exercise, knowing that I'm bound to hurt myself again.

Solution

There could be a number of reasons why you're injuring yourself whenever you exercise. With exercise, most injuries occur because of a lack of proper warm-up and stretching pre-exercise. Most people either skip the warm-up or stretch first—this is incorrect. Another cause of your injuries may be lack of flexibility. Your muscles must be warmed up before you do any quick-jerk movements, such as lifting weights or working out with weight machines. Medical statistics prove that the more flexible you become, the less your risk of injury. You could also be lifting with too much weight, or your form may not be correct when you are exercising.

It's important to note that these recurring injuries will go away only if you change the way you work out. Your form and technique are crucial to any type of exercise, but especially with weightlifting. Year in and year out, thousands of people injure themselves by exercising improperly or overdoing it. Most injuries can be avoided if you're flexible and your muscles are toned properly. Another cause of serious injury is coming back too soon from an existing ache or pain.

Learn to ease into your workouts, slowly building up intensity. With fitness, we are typically impatient and want it all—now! You should start out by exercising three times a week. Include a proper warm-up and stretch prior to your weightlifting, use lighter weights, and do more repetitions. Let your muscles get used to working before you increase the stress and torque on your joints. Check with a doctor or physical therapist familiar with your condition. He will be able to educate you about which exercises you should or should not be performing.

It's important for you to keep your confidence level up, even though at the moment you are unable to perform the exercises that you really would like to be doing. For example, if you have a "bad" back and the exercises you want to do would exacerbate your condition, that doesn't mean that you're never going to be able to do them. As you strengthen your abdominals and increase your range of motion and flexibility, chances are you'll eventually be able to start reintroducing them back into your regimen. Be patient, because if you play it smart, you can have it all. That's the key, and the number-one reason why most fitness enthusiasts never truly get over nagging injuries. They keep pounding and pounding, never allowing their injury to completely heal, rather than resting properly. I'm not advising you to stop exercising altogether. I'm saying that you need to learn how to work out differently without making your injury worse. That's difficult because we are not taught how to do that. So educate yourself and do the right thing to allow your injury to heal so that one day you'll be able to exercise and play golf "pain free."

I Can't Stick with It When I Travel.

I have to travel often for my profession. When I'm not traveling, my workouts are great. I'm consistent while I'm in town, but as soon as I hit the road, I find it difficult to keep up with my fitness regimen. I belong to a great health club, and I use free weights and weight machines. One of the problems I encounter that seems to get in the way of having a good workout while traveling is that none of the hotels have exercise equipment like my club at home. This is frustrating because I've never been able to reach a higher level of fitness, nor am I totally happy with the way I look.

Solution

Your problem can easily be fixed. Don't be surprised if the hotels you are staying at do not have the same equipment as your health club does. Most hotels do not have a great deal of space for workout equipment. Knowing that, you need to come up with a fitness routine that is not so machine-dependent. Equally important, you need to prepare yourself properly by practicing your travel routine before you go away. Do not wait to "try" your exercise regimen until you're on the road—you will fail. Performing your travel workout while you're at home, before you travel, serves a number of purposes: you'll see how long it takes you to complete your entire workout session so that you can make adjustments, if needed; you'll get used to working out without being so machine-dependent; you can memorize your routine so that you know exactly what to do; and most important, you'll realize that you don't really need to use all that machinery to maintain your fitness level. You have to learn to make the best of your situation. Instead of focusing on what you can't do, put your energies into what you *can* control. Pack a jump rope—jumping rope is one of the best exercises, and you can do it anywhere. Practice push-ups, chin-ups, and dips. Once you realize that you can still get in an effective workout while traveling, not only will you be relieved, but you'll stop your yo-yo syndrome and come back from your trips with your body looking and feeling its best.

I Feel Self-Conscious at the Gym.

Why is it that every time I go to the gym I feel totally lost and all alone? I am a very good golfer and never feel inadequate on the golf course, despite my lack of self-esteem about my body. Although I have received help from my club's staff, I'm still very intimidated and overwhelmed with all the complex fitness equipment (which I still don't understand how to use properly) and am petrified that everyone is watching and snickering at me behind my back. As a consequence, I've lost my interest, passion, and focus while I'm exercising at my health club.

Solution

Well, you certainly have a number of issues to address. First off, why are you paying money to go to a gym when you have not received the support and education that you obviously need and are seeking? Call the director of operations and make an appointment to discuss your concerns with her. Ask the gym staff if you can please be shown exactly how to use all the fitness equipment relevant to your fitness regimen, taking as much time as you need. Be very frank and honest with the staff that you don't appreciate their lack of commitment to you and your needs. If that doesn't work, do some research and find other gyms that better suit your needs. If there are none, I recommend that you work out at home and invest in some home fitness equipment. Either a stationary bike or a treadmill, along with a simple jump rope, a firm exercise mat, and a lightly weighted bar are all you really need. Hire a personal trainer for a couple of sessions to teach you some different workouts.

The fact that you're uncomfortable with your body sends out vibes to others, just as you would exude confidence if you felt better about yourself. I know plenty of men and women who are not great beauties, but project a certain aura and confidence. You happen to feel that way on the golf course, not at the health club. You are good at golf and you know what you're doing while playing the course; hence you don't experience anxiety on the links. With fitness, however, because you are unsure and hesitant, your focus is on others watching you rather than concentrating on the task at hand. As you learn more about what to do, and how to exercise properly, you will become so absorbed in exercising that even if you are being watched, you won't notice, or it won't bother you as much because you'll be more relaxed.

Remember, whatever constraints you may have—from physical to practical to emotional—you can become and stay fit. Look, we all—professional athletes included—have trouble from time to time motivating ourselves to exercise on a consistent basis. But the more you know about fitness, the more consistent you will be in your workout routine. The key is to identify and come to terms with what is truly keeping you from exercising. Once you've identified the cause for your inconsistency, you can come up with a game plan to make the necessary changes. And for every reason you come up with for not working out, remember, there are a thousand reasons why you can and should be exercising.

Above all, do not lose confidence and become discouraged. Think back and ask yourself, when was the last time you gave it your all and failed at an undertaking you sought to accomplish? I'll bet your success rate is directly related to the depth of your commitment, your determination to follow through, a sensible game plan, and most important, your passion and desire to succeed.

CHAPTER 6

Flexibility and Stretching

If you expect to hit the golf ball farther, you must increase your flexibility. It doesn't matter how strong you are if you cannot use all that strength. All of us can augment our flexibility by simply stretching a few minutes a day. The key to improving your flexibility and range of motion is to make sure you stretch before every golf swing and before each one of your workouts.

To gain the benefits of stretching and to improve your flexibility, you must warm up prior to stretching. Any aerobic exercise, such as walking, jogging, or biking, is adequate to get you warmed up. Warm up for at least ten minutes to get your body lubricated before you start stretching. A full-body stretch routine follows; this can be performed before your round of golf, before your workout, or at any time throughout the day. If you don't have enough time to warm up, make sure you walk around for at least a few minutes before attempting these stretches. Depending on the stretch you are performing, where applicable, hold each stretch between fifteen and sixty seconds. Do not bounce or jerk your body while stretching.

Basic Stretching Rules

- Stretch slowly and with control.
- Do not bounce.
- Stretch until you feel slight discomfort, not pain.
- Relax while you're stretching—your breath should be slow and rhythmic; don't hold your breath.
- Ease up on any stretch if you feel that it is too severe, and don't compare your flexibility to others'.
- Be patient—in time you will become more flexible and supple.
- You can stretch on any surface, including the ground, as long as you are comfortable. If you feel any discomfort, stretch on an exercise mat.

Please get your doctor or healthcare professional's clearance and permission to perform any of the following stretches and exercises. And be sure to refer to the DVD for instruction on the proper way to do each stretch.

The following stretches comprise your "stretch routine."

The Anatomy of a Golf Swing
The Upper Body

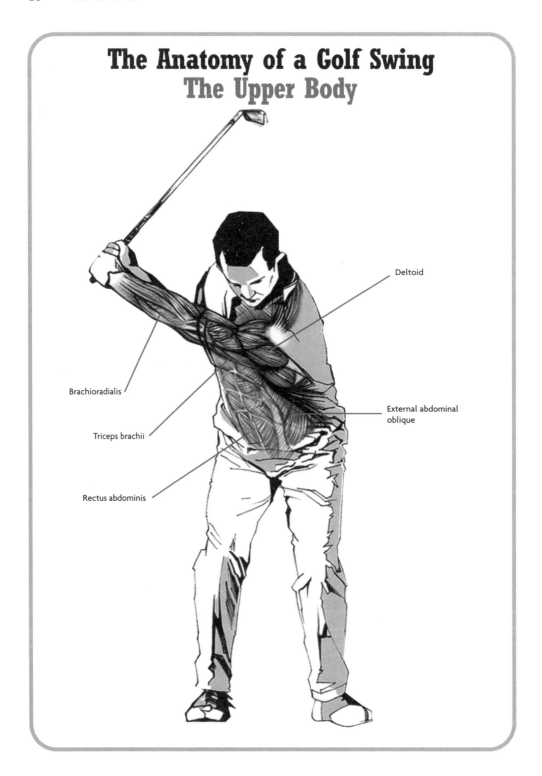

Deltoid

Brachioradialis

Triceps brachii

Rectus abdominis

External abdominal oblique

Upper Body Stretches

These upper body stretches allow you to draw the club back during your backswing, while keeping your left arm (right arm if you're left-handed) as straight as possible.

Arm Circles

With arms outstretched, slowly circle your arms backward for five revolutions, and then five revolutions forward. Try to create as big an arc as possible.

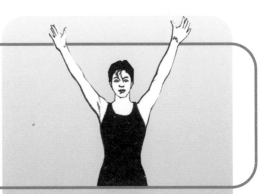

Triceps

With arms overhead, gently pull your left elbow behind your head with your right hand. Hold when you reach a comfortable stretch in the shoulder and upper back. Switch arms and repeat.

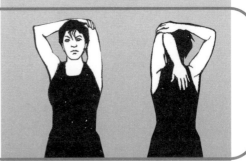

Shoulders and Chest

Grasp your hands behind your back, with palms facing each other. Slightly bend your knees and lift your arms up as you bend forward at the waist. Hold when you feel a comfortable stretch in the shoulders and chest.

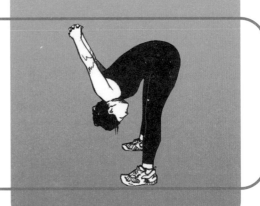

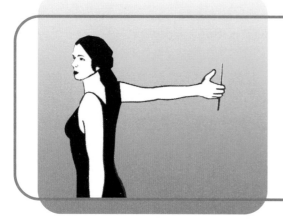

Arms, Upper Back, and Chest

While standing upright, reach behind you with your right arm, keeping it perfectly straight, and grasp onto a door molding or any other immovable object. Now, look over your left shoulder and hold the stretch. Switch to your left arm and repeat.

Stretches for the Torso, Lower Back, Hips, and Glutes

These core stretches allow you to turn properly during your backswing and help your entire midsection power through the ball.

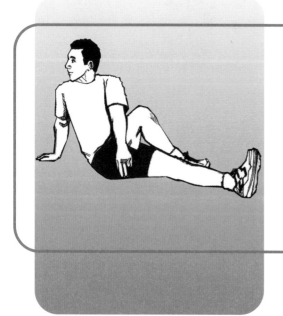

Spinal Twist #1

Sitting on the ground, keep your left leg straight, right arm behind you for support. Cross your right leg over your left knee and place your right foot outside your left knee. With your left hand or elbow on your right knee, slowly twist, and look over your right shoulder while simultaneously pulling your knee in the opposite direction; hold. You will feel pressure in the hip, side, and back. Repeat on the opposite side.

The Anatomy of a Golf Swing
Torso, Lower Back, Hips, and Glutes

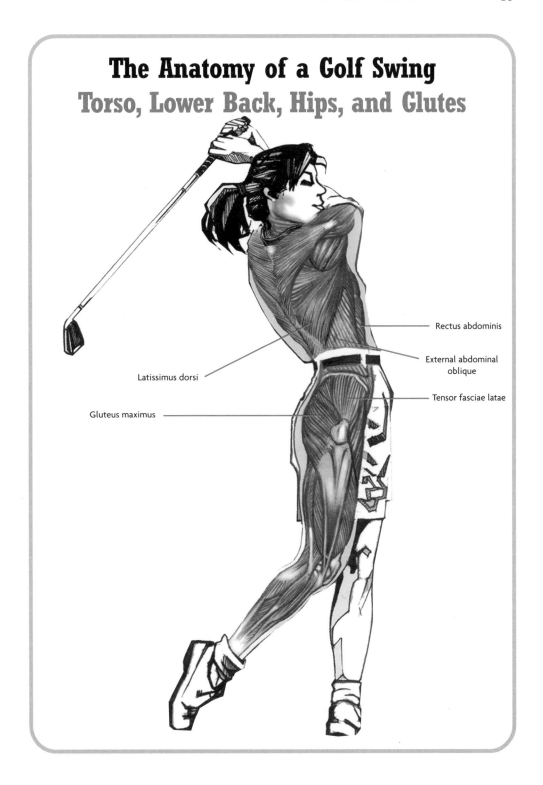

Rectus abdominis

External abdominal oblique

Latissimus dorsi

Tensor fasciae latae

Gluteus maximus

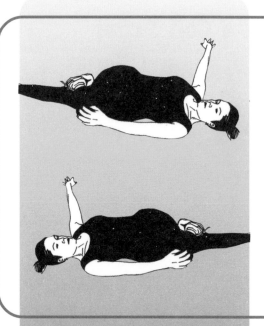

Spinal Twist #2

While lying on your back, bend your right leg, and hook your right toe behind your left knee, as shown. Keep your right arm out straight at a 90-degree angle to balance yourself. Take your left arm and hand and push down gently on your right knee while keeping your right shoulder blade touching the ground at all times. Turn your head to look toward your right hand while keeping your head resting on the ground at all times. Keep applying pressure with your left hand and try to get the right knee to touch the ground without the right shoulder blade leaving the ground. Repeat on the other side.

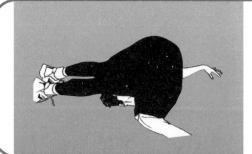

Roll Backs

While lying on your back, roll backward, and balance yourself on your upper shoulders, as shown. Try to extend your legs straight over your forehead and behind you as you hold the stretch.

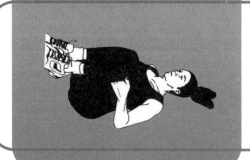

Knees to Chest

While lying on your back, bring both knees up toward your chest, as shown. Grab your right and left legs under your knees with each hand and pull your knees and legs in toward your chest.

The Anatomy of a Golf Swing
Lower Back, Groin, Legs, and Calves

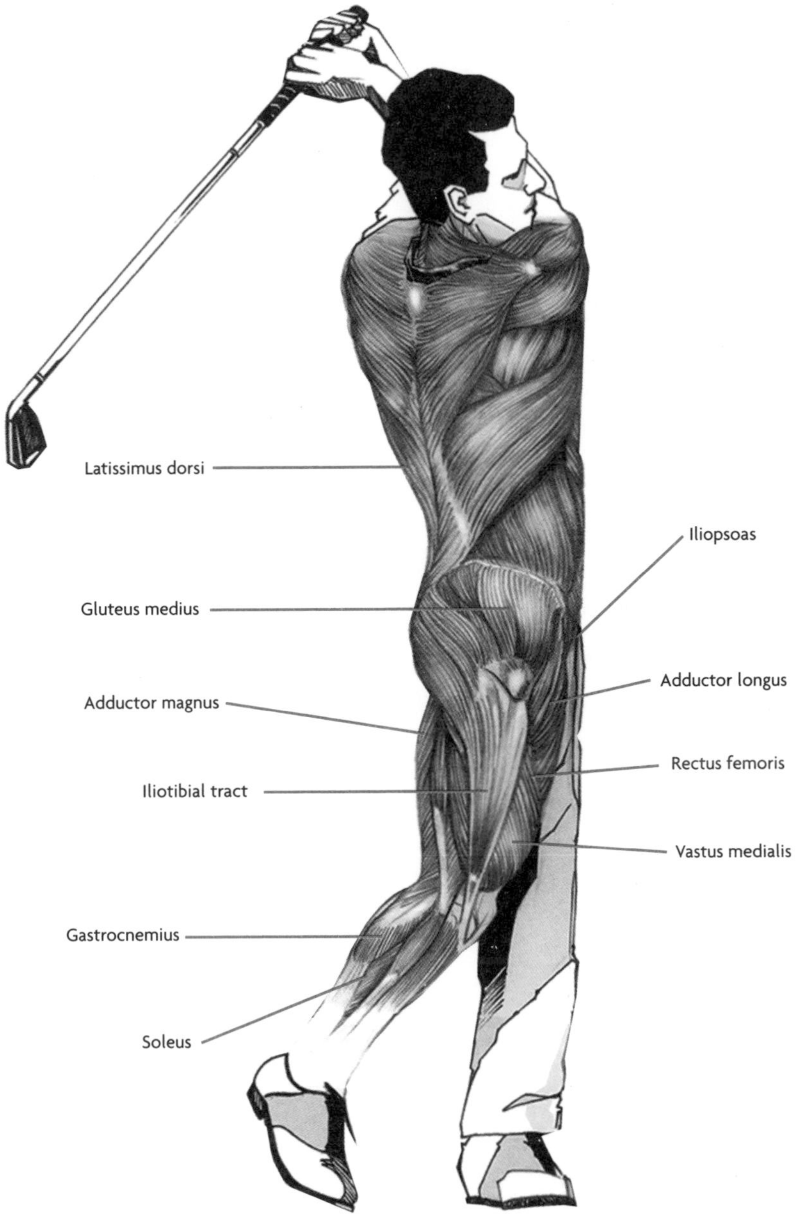

Latissimus dorsi

Iliopsoas

Gluteus medius

Adductor longus

Adductor magnus

Rectus femoris

Iliotibial tract

Vastus medialis

Gastrocnemius

Soleus

Stretches for the Lower Back, Groin, Legs, and Calves

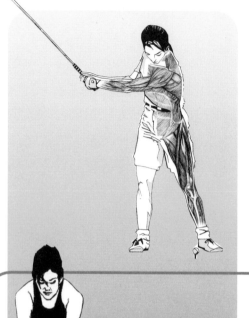

These stretches allow you to keep your lower body stable during your backswing and then transfer your weight to your left lower half (right lower half if you're a lefty) as you finish your golf swing.

Hamstrings—Legs Together

Sit down on the ground, with your legs straight, ankles flexed. Bend forward from your hips and reach out toward your toes and, based on your flexibility, grab onto your socks, shoelaces, or toes and hold the stretch. You will feel tension just behind the knees, upper calves, and in the lower back area.

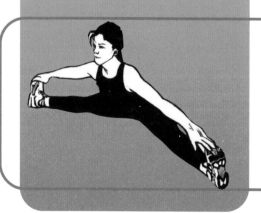

Hamstrings—Legs Apart

Sitting on the ground, with legs straight and apart, bend forward from the hips and reach toward your toes. Based on your flexibility, grab onto your toes or, if this is not possible, your socks or shoelaces.

Groin

In a sitting position on the ground, pull the soles of your feet together, and grab hold of your ankles. Gently pull your heels toward the groin area. Let your knees relax toward the floor, and gently press your elbows down on your knees to increase the stretch. If you are already flexible in this region of your body, grab your toes and lean forward as far as possible while keeping your back straight.

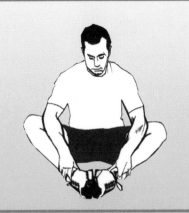

Quadriceps

Lie down on your left side or prop yourself up on your left elbow, as shown. Bend your right leg back and grab your right ankle with your right hand. Gently hold your right ankle and bring your right leg back toward your buttocks. Hold the position when you feel a comfortable stretch in the front of your thigh. Release slowly, roll over to your right side, and repeat.

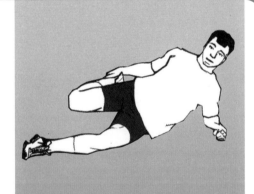

Calves #1

With hands and feet on the ground, make your body into a V shape. With both feet together, bend your right knee and press your left heel toward the ground, stretching your left calf. Repeat on the other side.

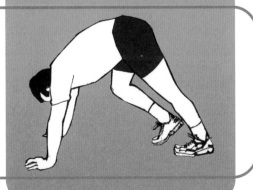

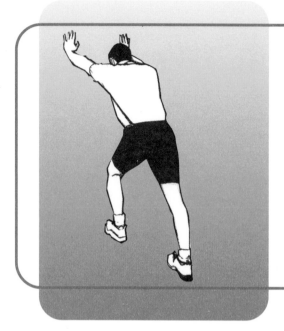

Calves #2

Stand arms-length away from a wall or another solid support. Lean on it with your hands placed shoulder-width apart. Bring your left foot forward, knee bent, while keeping the right leg straight. Lean toward the wall and keep your right heel on the ground while holding the stretch. Switch legs and repeat.

Other Trouble Spots

To loosen a tight neck, you might want to perform some simple neck circles clockwise 5 to 10 repetitions and counterclockwise 5 to 10 repetitions. To stretch your forearms, wrists, hands, and fingers, you can perform hand circles. You can also extend your arms straight in front of you and first clasp your hands with palms facing you, and then with palms facing away from you and hold the stretch. Lastly, as you monitor your exercise improvement, also monitor your increasing flexibility. If you are a little tight in a particular region of your body, you should stretch that area at the end of your workout or after you hit balls or play golf. It will make a big difference in your progress.

Advanced Stretches and Calisthenics

The following stretches and calisthenics can be performed in conjunction with the previous stretches or on their own. Make sure, though, that you are properly warmed up before your perform any of the exercises illustrated below.

Achilles Tendon and Hamstrings

Bend over and place your hands out in front of you on the ground with your legs straight. Flex your ankles and lean back on your heels while balancing yourself on your fingers. Hold the stretch in this position.

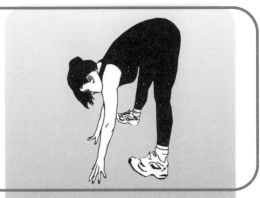

Chest, Shoulders, and Quadriceps

Lying on your stomach, reach behind and grab the top of each foot with each hand, as shown. Lift your chest off the ground and hold.

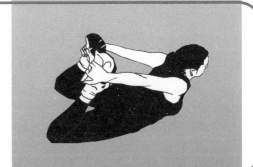

Chest Tilts

While lying on your stomach with your arms by your sides, lift your chest off the ground as far as possible and hold. Keep your thighs on the ground to help maintain your balance and keep your head up the entire time you hold the position.

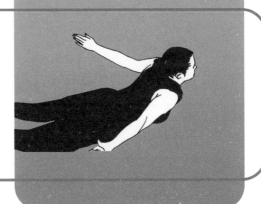

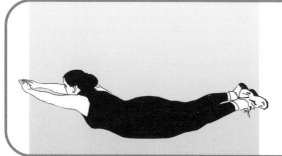

Diver Position

Lying on your stomach, straighten and bring your arms together and clasp your hands. Bring your legs together and point your toes. Lift your chest and your legs off the ground simultaneously and hold.

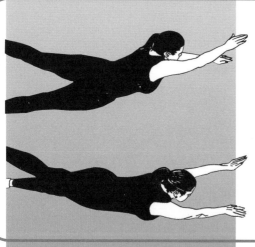

Opposite Arms and Legs

Lying on your stomach, bring your arms in front of your body and fully extend your legs behind you. Lift your left leg off the ground as you lift your right arm and hold this position. To work the opposite arm and leg, switch to lifting your right leg and left arm off the ground simultaneously.

Fitness Prescriptions for Weight Loss

In order to lose weight and/or sustain weight loss, you must practice proper exercise and have a deficit in your caloric intake. If you don't do both, the result will be failure. Sure, you might initially lose some weight through extreme dieting or other means but, in the long run, you will never achieve your weight loss goals and maintain your sought-after weight. The only people I've worked with over the years who have not lost the weight they wanted were those who ignored these two principles.

That being said, proper exercise—how you exercise—has a lot to do with whether you see immediate results, which in turn will keep you motivated. The types of exercises you perform will dictate how much fat you burn, your metabolic rate, and how much food you eat, among other things. You may have heard that if you have more muscle, you will burn more fat. In theory, this is true, but this is often interpreted to mean that you need to lift weights to have more muscle. This is not accurate—lifting weights does not guarantee that you will raise your Basal Metabolic Rate (the calories your

body uses in a day). The deciding factor in raising your BMR is how hard you work (intensity), not the type of exercises you perform. You don't need to lift weights to have a healthy body ratio (the amount of lean muscle and body fat, based on your body weight). For instance, ballerinas often don't lift any weights, yet are slim and lithe. Similarly, swimmers, divers, and marathon runners tend to be on the slim side and in general do not lift weights. It is more a function of how hard you exercise as opposed to the type of exercise you perform that dictates your body ratio. As a nonathlete, if you burn more fat (with aerobic exercise and light weights), you will have a better body ratio because your body-fat percentage will be less than before you began exercising; hence, you will have a higher ratio of muscle to fat.

There are two other fallacies that need to be cleared up before you start exercising for weight loss. We often hear that muscle weighs more than fat. This is actually a misleading statement. What people mean to say is that, per square inch, muscle is denser than fat and, therefore, per square inch, weighs more than fat. That's why people who have a high fat content look like they weigh more than they actually do and those who are more muscular and defined appear to weigh less than they actually do. To illustrate this visually, a pound of fat is about the size of your fist and a pound of muscle is about the size of a silver dollar. Since fat occupies approximately three times the area of muscle, the more fat you lose, the smaller you look. That's why one person may look trimmer than another but they may both register the same weight on the scale.

The other misconception is that fat can be converted to muscle. Unfortunately, fat cannot be converted to muscle, and, conversely, muscle does not turn to fat. So, in reality, you cannot firm the fat on the back of your arms, or anywhere else on your body. You can, however, lose the fat on your body and build muscle underneath the fat, but you need to make sure when you exercise for weight loss that the rate at which you burn fat is greater than the rate at which you build muscle. The more fat you have in a region of your body and the more muscle you build underneath it, the bigger that region of your body becomes.

Exercising for Weight Loss

Here are some guidelines to consider as you plan your weight loss fitness regimen:

- Work out a minimum of three to four days a week.

- Work up to thirty to forty minutes of continuous aerobic exercise.

- Don't allow more than two days to elapse between exercising.

- On days when you fall off your eating plan or have overeaten, make sure you exercise the following day.

- The majority of your workout time (duration) should be aerobic (not anaerobic).

- Use light weights and high reps for all exercises. (Repetitions, or "reps," are the number of times you actually perform an exercise.)

- Use light to moderate resistance/tension on all aerobic-type exercises.

- As you lose weight and are closer to your "ideal" body weight, you can increase your resistance/tension and weights for all exercises.

- Instead of focusing on building more muscle, concentrate on burning fat. By doing so, you will have a healthier body ratio of muscle to fat and less overall mass.

- As you become more aerobically fit, you need to keep increasing the intensity of your workout to ensure that you are burning enough calories.

- If you can't do all the repetitions for an given exercise, don't skip the exercise. Simply do what you can. Keep track and eventually you will be able to do the recommended repetitions plus more!

Each of the exercise prescriptions to follow is designed to be performed in your home, at any gym, or even while you're traveling. If you are a beginner exerciser, first watch the enclosed DVD so that you can become more confident about doing the exercises with proper form, alignment, and technique. The DVD demonstrates how the stretches and exercises should be performed. Please follow the fitness prescriptions outlined here and, when needed, watch the DVD to see how a particular exercise movement is properly executed.

Fitness Equipment for Weight Loss

You want to keep your fitness program as simple as possible, so your exercise equipment should be easy to use, and the instructions for use easy to understand. Make sure that you can perform all the exercises no matter where you are because consistency and frequency are the keys to your success! Although you may use any piece of aerobic fitness equipment for the aerobic portion of your workouts, I highly recommend that you use a recumbent stationary bike. It's easy on your back and knees and it's comfortable, so you'll want to stick with your exercise regimen.

Choose one or more of the following pieces of aerobic equipment: a recumbent or upright stationary bike, a treadmill, an elliptical machine, a cross-trainer, or, if you don't have access to any equipment, walk or jog instead.

You may also need:

- **A firm exercise mat for abdominal exercises**
- **A lightweight (2–4-lb.) collapsible aerobic bar for calisthenics and upper body exercises**
- **For men, an 8–10-lb. weighted bar for upper body exercises**
- **A lightweight speed jump rope**

Your workouts are designed to help you take weight off and also firm and tone your body. As you get within ten to fifteen pounds of your "ideal weight," you may switch over to the endurance workouts detailed in chapter 8.

If you need a break at any time during your exercise regimen, you can get on a stationary bike or any other piece of aerobic equipment or walk for one to three minutes to allow your heart rate to come down safely before you resume. Also, if you want to pay more attention to either your upper body, your midsection, or your lower body, you can perform more repetitions or do an extra set of exercises that target that region.

If you can perform more repetitions with any exercise, please go ahead and do so. If not, keep track of how many repetitions you do for all your exercises, and as you increase your fitness level you will be able to comfortably increase the number of repetitions you perform. Try to add one to two repetitions for each exercise every two to three weeks, working up to fifty to sixty repetitions for each exercise. Work up to ten to twenty minutes of continuous jumping rope.

While exercising, if you feel that these workouts are not challenging enough for you, add repetitions—not weight or tension/resistance—or increase duration or speed.

Before you start any fitness plan, consult your healthcare professional or doctor for approval.

How to Jump Rope

Many people think that jumping rope is bad on your knees or causes injuries, but if you follow these guidelines, it is a safe and highly effective exercise.

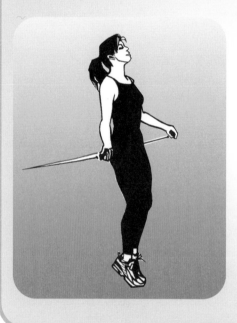

- Make sure you jump on a surface that has some give to it, such as a wooden floor, short grass, or a rubberized track or tennis court. *Do not* jump on asphalt or cement.

- Practice swinging the rope overhead without jumping, forming a loop.

- Move your forearms in time with your feet.

- Jump just high enough for the rope to pass under your feet (one inch off the ground). Jump with both feet at once. (Jumping higher than one inch will cause unnecessary stress to the legs, increasing the potential for injury.)

- The rope should hit the ground about one foot in front of your feet with each revolution.

   Caution: avoid double jumping. Your workout will not be as effective. After each jump the rope should pass under your feet.

Program A: Full Body Exercise Regimen

Frequency: 3 days a week, every other day.
Duration: 50 to 60 minutes, depending on your current level of fitness.

Warm-up and aerobic segment

Do one of the following for 30 minutes:

- Bike with light tension/resistance at 80+ rpm or 12+ mph.
- Walk at 3.5+ mph or slow jog at 5.0 mph with no hills or incline.
- If you are using an elliptical machine or cross-trainer, do moderate to high speed with light resistance and/or incline.

Stretch

Hold each of the following stretches for 30 to 60 seconds. To aid you with your stretches and to help you memorize your stretch routine, watch the DVD.

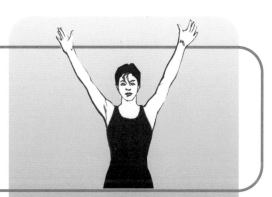

Arm Circles

With arms outstretched, slowly circle your arms backward for five revolutions, and then five revolutions forward. Try to create as big an arc as possible.

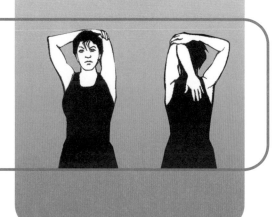

Triceps

With arms overhead, gently pull your left elbow behind your head with your right hand. Hold when you reach a comfortable stretch in the shoulder and upper back. Switch arms and repeat.

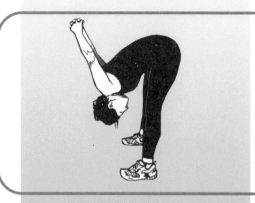

Shoulders and Chest

Grasp your hands behind your back, with palms facing each other. Slightly bend your knees and lift your arms up as you bend forward at the waist. Hold when you feel a comfortable stretch in the shoulders and chest.

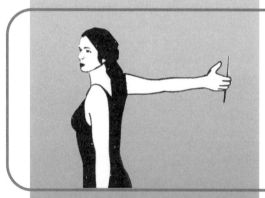

Arms, Upper Back, and Chest

While standing upright, reach behind you with your right arm, keeping it perfectly straight, and grasp onto a door molding or any other immovable object. Now, look over your opposite shoulder and hold the stretch. Switch to your left arm and repeat.

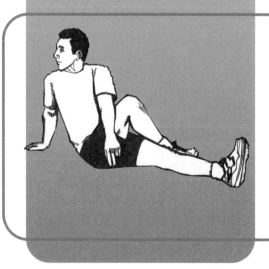

Spinal Twist #1

Sitting on the ground, keep your left leg straight, right arm behind you for support. Cross your right leg over your left knee and place your right foot outside your left knee. With your left hand or elbow on your right knee, slowly twist, and look over your right shoulder while simultaneously pulling your knee in the opposite direction; hold. You will feel pressure in the hip, side, and back. Repeat on the opposite side.

Spinal Twist #2

While lying on your back, bend your right leg, and hook your right toe behind your left knee, as shown. Keep your right arm out straight at a 90-degree angle to balance yourself. Take your left arm and hand and push down gently on your right knee while keeping your right shoulder blade touching the ground at all times. Turn your head to look toward your right hand while keeping your head resting on the ground at all times. Keep applying pressure with your left hand and try to get the right knee to touch the ground without the right shoulder blade leaving the ground. Repeat on the other side.

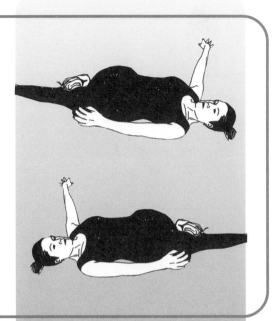

Roll Backs

While lying on your back, roll backward, and balance yourself on your upper shoulders, as shown. Try to extend your legs straight over your forehead and behind you as you hold the stretch.

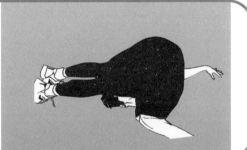

Knees to Chest

While lying on your back, bring both knees up toward your chest, as shown. Grab your right and left legs under your knees with each hand and pull your knees and legs in toward your chest.

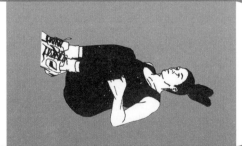

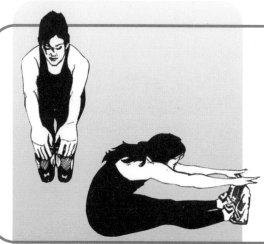

Hamstrings—Legs Together

Sit down on the ground with your legs straight, ankles flexed. Bend forward from your hips and reach out toward your toes and, based on your flexibility, grab onto your socks, shoelaces, or toes and hold the stretch. You will feel tension just behind the knees, upper calves, and in the lower back area.

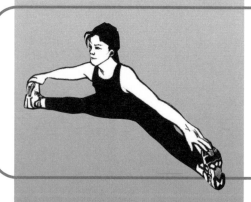

Hamstrings—Legs Apart

Sitting on the ground, with legs straight and apart, bend forward from the hips and reach toward your toes. Based on your flexibility, grab onto your toes or, if this is not possible, your socks or shoelaces.

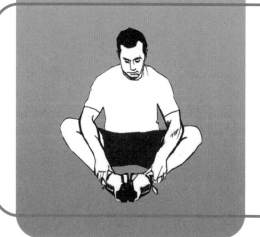

Groin

In a sitting position, pull the soles of your feet together, and grab hold of your ankles. Gently pull your heels toward the groin area. Let your knees relax toward the floor, and gently press your elbows down on your knees to increase the stretch. If you are already flexible in this region of your body, grab your toes and lean forward as far as possible while keeping your back straight.

Quadriceps

Lie down on your left side and prop your-self up on your left elbow, as shown. Bend your right leg back and grab your right ankle with your right hand. Gently hold your right ankle and bring your leg back toward your buttocks. Hold the position when you feel a comfortable stretch in the front of your thigh. Release slowly, roll over to your right side, and repeat.

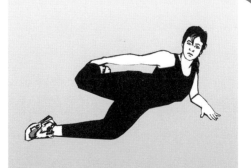

Calves #1

With hands and feet on the ground, make your body into a V shape. With both feet together, bend your right knee and press your left heel toward the ground, stretching your left calf. Repeat on the other side.

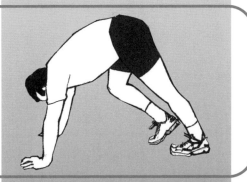

Calves #2

Stand arms-length away from a wall or another solid support. Lean on it with your hands placed shoulder-width apart. Bring your left foot forward, knee bent, while keeping the right leg straight. Lean toward the wall and keep your right heel on the ground while holding the stretch. Switch legs and repeat.

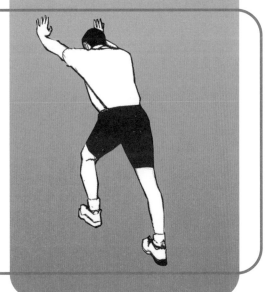

Workload

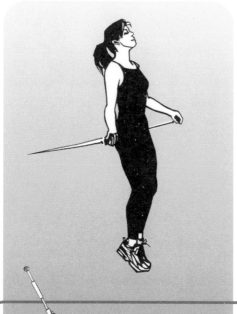

Aerobic Segment

Jump rope for 1 minute, then spend 3 minutes biking, walking, jogging, or using any aerobic equipment of your choice—with moderate intensity. If you cannot jump rope, then perform 5 minutes on your choice of aerobic equipment.

Please note: you may also perform side benders after your aerobic segment or at any time during your workout to catch your breath and/or work on your obliques and range of motion.

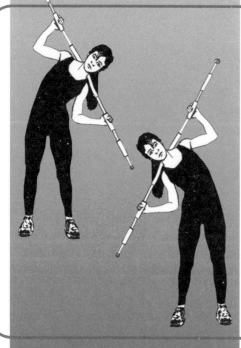

Side Benders

While standing upright, legs hip-width apart, place the aerobic bar on your neck, as shown. Bend to the left side as far as possible without moving your hips or legs. Maintain your stability. Now bend back to the right side as far as possible. Do not stop in the middle. Keep repeating the movement back and forth at a slow pace until you've caught your breath.

To keep from building up too much muscle under the fat, do not use more than a 4-lb. aerobic bar while performing side benders. As you lose weight, increase the weight of the bar as you perform side benders.

Abdominals/Hips and Legs

These exercises help strengthen your entire core region and your hips, and help trim and tone your legs.

To be performed on a firm exercise mat.

Sit-Ups *(Beginner)*

20 to 40 reps

Lie on your back with your knees bent, feet flat on the floor with heels up against your mat, with your hands clasped behind the midsection of your neck. Slowly raise your shoulder blades up a few inches while bringing your chest toward your knees. Exhale while curling up. Slowly lower your body to the starting position and repeat.

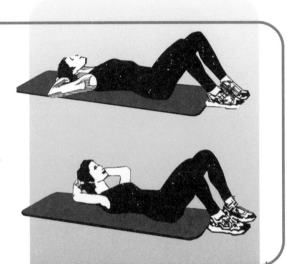

Sit-Ups *(Intermediate)*

20 to 40 reps

Lie on your back with your knees bent, feet flat on the floor with heels up against your mat, your thumbs clasped with your arms fully extended, as shown. Slowly raise your arms (keep them straight) toward your knees and perform a full sit-up. Exhale while sitting up. Slowly lower your body to the starting position and repeat.

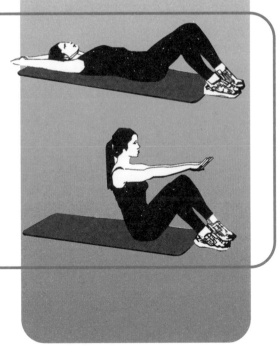

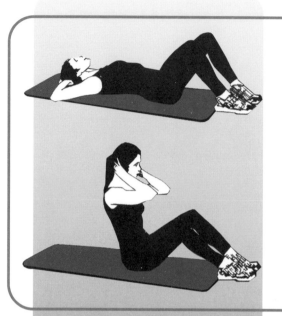

Sit-Ups *(Advanced)*

20 to 40 reps

Lie on your back with your knees bent, feet flat on the floor with heels up against your mat, your hands on your ears, as shown. Slowly raise your body all the way up, bringing your elbows toward your knees. Exhale while sitting up. Slowly lower your body to the starting position as you inhale and repeat.

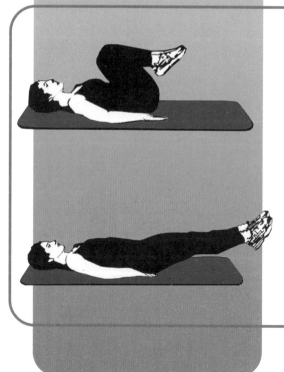

Leg-Outs

20 reps, rest 30 seconds, then repeat 20 reps

Lying on your back, with your hands under your buttocks, palms down, bring both knees in toward your chest. Slowly straighten your legs out with toes pointed and repeat. Inhale while bringing your knees toward your chest; exhale as you straighten your legs. Beginners should straighten their legs out at a higher angle. As you get stronger, try to bring your legs lower (about two inches from the ground) while straightening them.

Please note: as your back and abs get stronger, you can move your hands from under your buttocks to behind your neck to intensify the exercise.

Alternates

20 reps, rest 30 seconds, then do another 20 reps

Lie on your back with your hands under your buttocks, palms down, or clasped behind your neck, as shown, legs straight, and toes pointed. Raise your right leg to a 90-degree angle; your left leg stays on the floor. Pressing the small of your back into the floor, lower your right leg as you simultaneously lift your left leg to a 90-degree angle. Continuously repeat this scissoring motion.

Please note: as your back and abs get stronger, you can move your hands from under your buttocks to behind your neck to intensify the exercise.

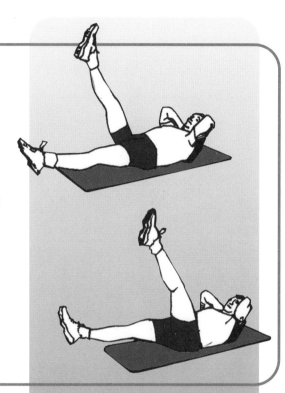

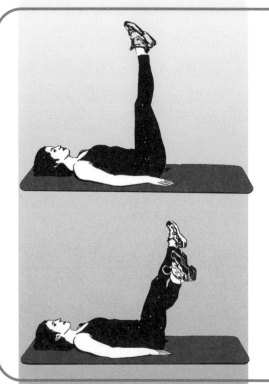

Vertical Scissors

**20 reps, rest 30 seconds,
then do another 20 reps**

Lie on your back, hands at your sides or next to or under your buttocks, with palms facing down. Raise both legs to a 90-degree angle. Pressing your back into the floor and with toes pointed and legs straight, slowly open your legs as wide as possible and then bring them back together while exhaling, keeping your toes pointed and your legs straight as you repeat the exercise.

Please note: if you have poor hamstring flexibility, do not attempt this exercise until you have improved that flexibility. As you get stronger, you can intensify this exercise by extending your arms straight out at a 90-degree angle with palms facing down to help maintain your balance.

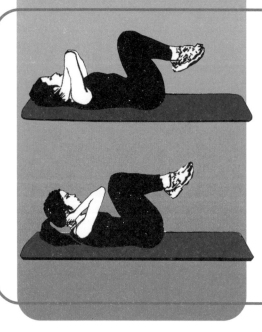

Elbows to Knees

20 reps

Lying on your back, raise your knees and feet toward your chest in a tucked position. Clasp your hands at the base of your neck. Gently curl your upper body, bringing your elbows toward your knees while exhaling. Slowly lower your back and shoulders to the mat while inhaling and repeat. Keep your lower body motionless throughout the entire movement.

Please note: if you cannot touch your elbows to your knees, reach as far as possible. As you increase your hamstring flexibility, you will be able to touch your elbows to your knees.

Aerobic Segment

Jump rope for 1 minute, then spend 3 minutes biking, walking, jogging, or using any aerobic equipment of your choice—with moderate intensity. If you cannot jump rope, then perform 5 minutes on your choice of aerobic equipment.

Please note: you may also perform side benders after your aerobic segment or at any time during your workout to catch your breath and/or work on your obliques and range of motion.

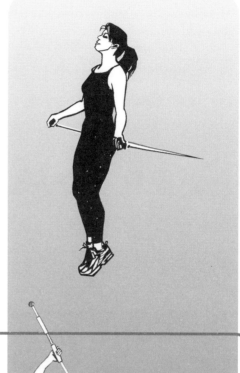

Side Benders

While standing upright, legs hip-width apart, place the aerobic bar on your neck, as shown. Bend to the left side as far as possible without moving your hips or legs. Maintain your stability. Now bend back to the right side as far as possible. Do not stop in the middle. Keep repeating the movement back and forth at a slow pace until you've caught your breath.

To keep from building up too much muscle under the fat, do not use more than a 4-lb. aerobic bar while performing side benders. As you lose weight, increase the weight of the bar as you perform side benders.

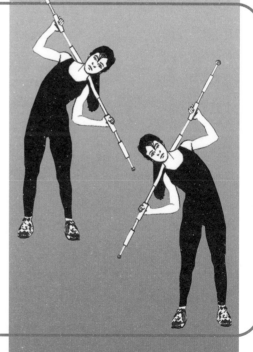

Legs/Hips

These exercises help slim and tone your inner and outer thighs, and help strengthen your calves, and improve balance.

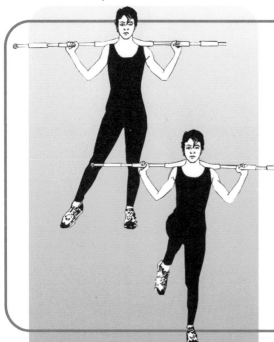

Standing Knee to Opposite Chest

20 to 30 reps

Rest the aerobic bar on your neck across your shoulders, with your feet hip-width apart. Transfer all your weight to your left leg. Raise your right knee up toward the left side of your chest to at least waist level, while exhaling. Lower your right toe to the starting position, touching the ground while keeping your weight on your left leg throughout the entire movement. Keep your back and aerobic bar completely straight without moving during the entire exercise. Perform all reps on one leg at a time and then switch legs and repeat.

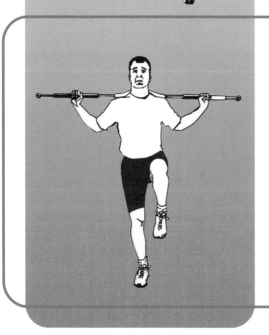

March in Place

50 to 60 reps

Rest the aerobic bar across your shoulders with your feet hip-width apart and balance yourself up on your toes. Raise your left knee straight up to at least waist level, aiming toward your chest. Keep your back straight and your abdominals contracted. Lower your left leg/foot to the starting position and switch to raising your right knee. Alternate legs rhythmically throughout the entire exercise. While marching in place, try to keep up on your toes while performing all the repetitions—try not to let your heels touch the ground at any time.

L-Kicks

20 to 30 reps

Hold the aerobic bar upright with your left hand and place your right hand on your waist. Start by raising your right leg in front of you, toe pointed, trying to get it to waist level, keeping it as straight as possible without leaning your weight on the bar. Then return to the starting position, lightly touching the ground. Now raise the right leg out to the side as high as possible, toe pointed, keeping it as straight as possible without leaning your weight on the bar. Return to the starting position and repeat the entire exercise. After you have completed all of your repetitions with your right leg, switch legs, and repeat with your left leg while holding the aerobic bar with your right hand.

Please note: the exercises on these two pages should be done in the following order: Standing Knee to Opposite Chest, then L-Kicks, then March in Place, as performed on the DVD.

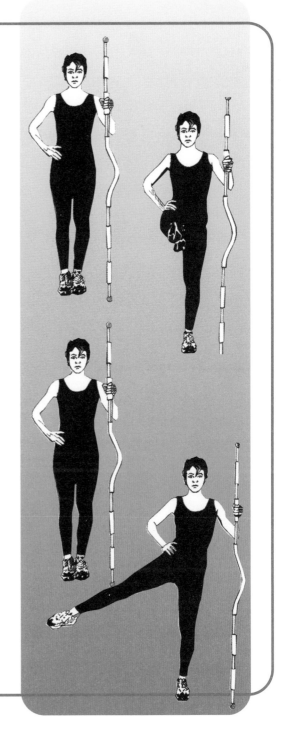

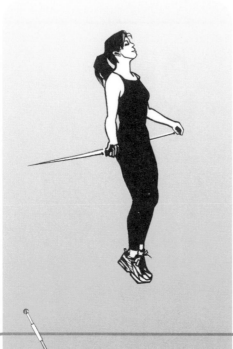

Aerobic Segment

Jump rope for 1 minute, then spend 3 minutes biking, walking, jogging, or using any aerobic equipment of your choice—with moderate intensity. If you cannot jump rope, then perform 5 minutes on your choice of aerobic equipment.

Please note: you may also perform side benders after your aerobic segment or at any time during your workout to catch your breath and/or work on your obliques and range of motion.

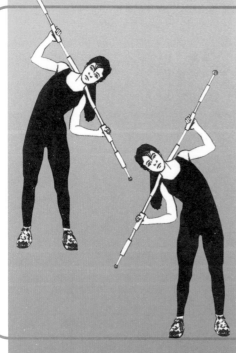

Side Benders

While standing upright, legs hip-width apart, place the aerobic bar on your neck, as shown. Bend to the left side as far as possible without moving your hips or legs. Maintain your stability. Now bend back to the right side as far as possible. Do not stop in the middle. Keep repeating the movement back and forth at a slow pace until you've caught your breath.

To keep from building up too much muscle under the fat, do not use more than a 4-lb. aerobic bar while performing side benders. As you lose weight, increase the weight of the bar as you perform side benders.

Upper Body Exercises

These exercises help tone your upper body and strengthen your arms.
To be performed with a 4-lb. aerobic bar for women and an 8–10-lb. weighted bar for men.

Push-Outs

25 to 35 reps

Keep your back straight, knees slightly bent, arms straight, and your feet just wider than shoulder-width apart. Grip the bar, palms facing down, just wider than shoulder width. Raise the bar up just above your chest line with your elbows up and wrists firm. Extend your arms straight out, holding the bar level above your chest and exhale. While inhaling, let your arms drop down to the front of your thighs, keeping your arms straight. Bring the bar back to the starting position and repeat. Keep your lower body aligned and still throughout the entire exercise. Maintain a moderate speed throughout the movement.

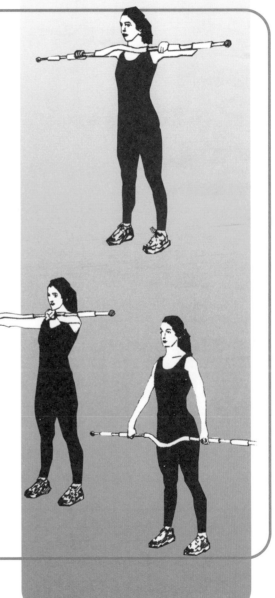

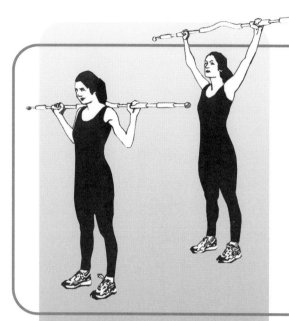

Behind-Neck Press

30 to 40 reps

Grip the bar slightly wider than shoulder width and place it behind your neck and shoulders. Keep your back straight, knees slightly bent, and your feet just wider than hip-width apart. Fully extend your arms upward and raise the bar straight up behind your neck while exhaling. Bend your arms and slowly return the bar to the back of your neck while inhaling and repeat. Make sure you keep the bar as close as possible to the back of your head to avoid neck discomfort.

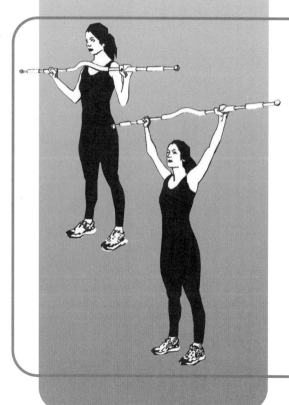

Front Press

30 to 40 reps

Keep your back straight, knees slightly bent, and feet shoulder-width apart. Grip the bar just past shoulder width and rest the bar across the top of your chest. Fully extend your arms upward and raise the bar straight up while exhaling. Bend your arms and slowly return the bar to the top of your chest while inhaling and repeat. Maintain a moderate speed throughout the entire movement.

Bent-Over Rows

30 to 40 reps

Place the bar on the ground in front of you, knees slightly bent and hands wider than shoulder-width apart, and bend over with your torso parallel to the floor. Pull the bar straight up toward the lower part of your chest while exhaling. Keeping your lower body still throughout the entire exercise, lower the bar to the starting position while inhaling. Keep your head up and your back as straight as possible. This can also be done with a narrow grip. Maintain a moderate speed throughout the entire movement.

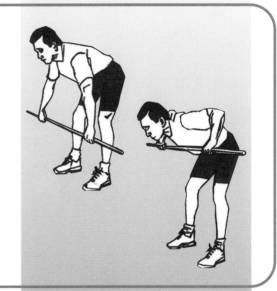

Upright Rows

35 to 45 reps

Keep your back straight, knees slightly bent, and feet hip-width apart. Grip the bar, palms facing down, 6 to 8 inches apart. Hold the bar with your arms fully extended at the front of your thighs. Slowly raise the bar up to your chin, keeping your elbows at or above bar level while exhaling. Return to the starting position while inhaling and repeat. You can also perform this exercise with a wide grip. Maintain a moderate speed throughout the entire movement.

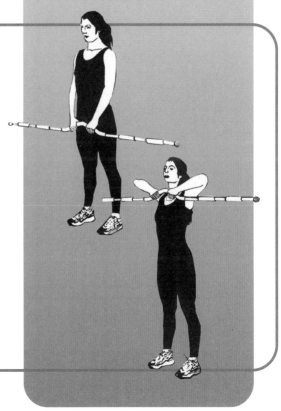

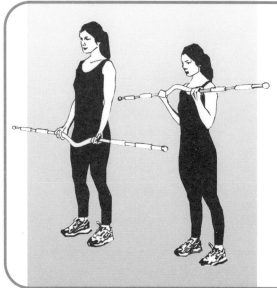

Curls

35 to 45 reps

Keep your back straight, knees slightly bent, and feet hip-width apart. Grip the bar, palms facing up and shoulder-width apart. Hold the bar with your arms fully extended at the front of your thighs. Keeping your elbows stationary and your wrists firm, curl the bar up to your chest while exhaling. Slowly extend your arms and return the bar to the starting position while inhaling and repeat. This exercise can be done with either a narrow or a wide grip. Maintain a moderate speed throughout the entire movement.

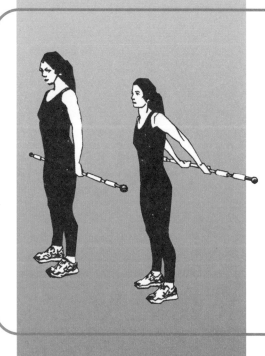

Kick-Backs

20 to 30 reps

Keep your back straight, knees slightly bent, and feet hip-width apart. Grip the bar with arms fully extended at the buttocks, palms facing outward about shoulder-width apart. Keeping your elbows stationary and wrists firm, lift the bar away from your buttocks as far as possible while exhaling. Keeping your arms straight, lower the bar to your buttocks while inhaling and repeat. Maintain a moderate speed throughout the entire movement.

Advanced Kick-Backs

10 to 20 reps

Keep your back straight, knees slightly bent, and feet hip-width apart. Grip the bar with your arms fully extended at the buttocks, palms facing outward, about shoulder-width apart. Keeping your wrists firm, bend your elbows while lifting the bar up to your lower back and then lift the bar away from your buttocks as far as possible while exhaling. Keeping your arms straight, lower the bar to the buttocks while inhaling and repeat. Maintain a moderate speed throughout the entire movement.

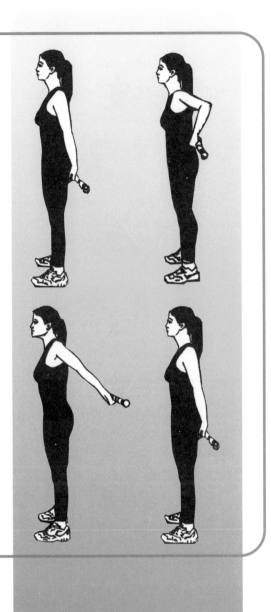

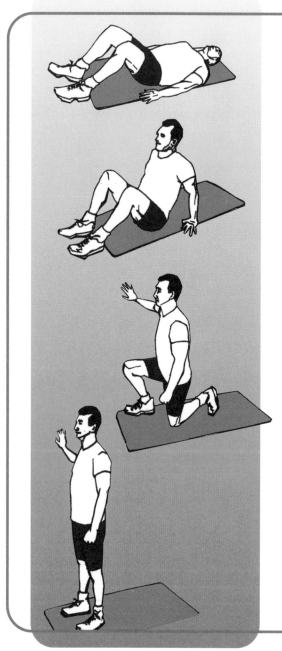

Stand-Ups

This exercise helps burn fat throughout the body and improves balance.

5 to 10 reps

Lie on your back with your knees bent and your heels on the floor, and press yourself up into a seated position while keeping your knees bent. Lift your body and come onto your hands and knees and place your right foot flat on the floor with your weight on your left knee, keeping your back straight. Place your right hand on an immovable object such as a wall as you lift your body up to a standing position. Return to the starting position and repeat the exercise. You may want to split up the reps by doing 5 or so on your right side and 5 or so on your left side, so as not to favor one side or the other.

Cool-down

Three minutes of easy biking or walking leisurely.

Program B: Aerobic/Abs Regimen

Frequency: 2 to 3 days a week.
Duration: 40 to 50 minutes, depending on your current level of fitness.

Warm-up and aerobic segment

Do one of the following for 30 to 40 minutes:

- Bike with light tension/resistance at 80+ rpm or 12+ mph.

- Walk at 3.5+ mph or slow jog at 5.0 mph with no hills or incline.

- If you are using an elliptical trainer or a cross-trainer, do moderate to high speed with light resistance and/or incline.

Please note: you should not perform program **A** two days in a row. You can, however, perform program **B** on successive days. Also, if you want to rest or need a day off, skip program **B**, not program **A**, whenever possible.

Stretch

Hold each stretch for 30 to 60 seconds. To aid you with your stretches and to help you memorize your stretch routine, watch the DVD.

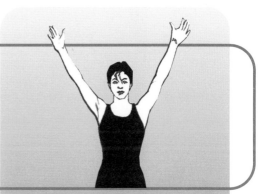

Arm Circles

With arms outstretched, slowly circle your arms backward for five revolutions, and then five revolutions forward. Try to create as big an arc as possible.

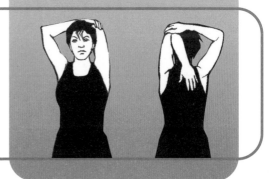

Triceps

With arms overhead, gently pull your left elbow behind your head with your right hand. Hold when you reach a comfortable stretch in the shoulder and upper back. Switch arms and repeat.

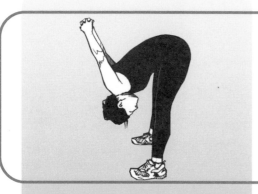

Shoulders and Chest

Grasp your hands behind your back, with palms facing each other. Slightly bend your knees and lift your arms up as you bend forward at the waist. Hold when you feel a comfortable stretch in the shoulders and chest.

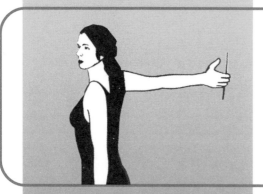

Arms, Upper Back, and Chest

While standing upright, reach behind you with your right arm, keeping it perfectly straight, and grasp onto a door molding or any other immovable object. Now look over your left shoulder and hold the stretch. Switch to your left arm and repeat.

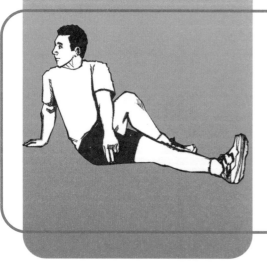

Spinal Twist #1

Sitting on the ground, keep your left leg straight, right arm behind you for support. Cross your right leg over your left knee and place your right foot outside your left knee. With your left hand or elbow on your right knee, slowly twist, and look over your right shoulder while simultaneously pulling your knee in the opposite direction; hold. You will feel pressure in the hip, side, and back. Repeat on the opposite side.

Spinal Twist #2

While lying on your back, bend your right leg, and hook your right toe behind your left knee, as shown. Keep your right arm out straight at a 90-degree angle to maintain your balance. Take your left arm and hand and push down gently on your right knee while keeping your right shoulder blade flat on the ground at all times. Turn your head to look toward your right hand while keeping your head resting on the ground at all times. Keep applying pressure with your left hand and try to get the right knee to touch the ground without the right shoulder blade leaving the ground. Repeat on the other side.

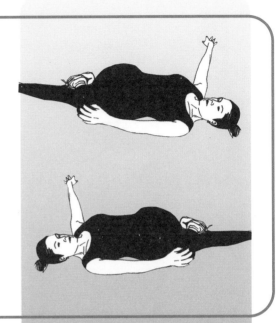

Roll Backs

While lying on your back, roll backward, and balance yourself on your upper shoulders, as shown. Try to extend your legs straight over your forehead and behind you as you hold the stretch.

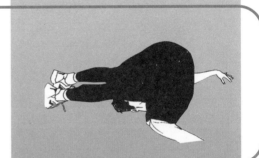

Knees to Chest

While lying on your back, bring both knees up toward your chest, as shown. Grab your right and left legs under your knees with each hand and pull your knees and legs in toward your chest.

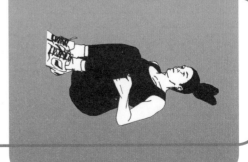

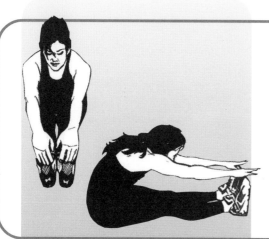

Hamstrings—Legs Together

Sit down on the ground with your legs straight, ankles flexed. Bend forward from your hips and reach out toward your toes. Based on your flexibility, grab onto your socks, shoelaces, or toes and hold the stretch. You will feel tension just behind the knees, upper calves, and in the lower back area.

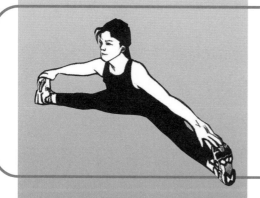

Hamstrings—Legs Apart

Sitting on the ground, with legs straight and apart, bend forward from the hips and reach toward your toes. Based on your flexibility, grab onto your toes or, if this is not possible, your socks or shoelaces.

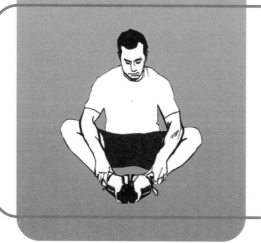

Groin

In a sitting position, pull the soles of your feet together, and grab hold of your ankles. Gently pull your heels toward the groin area. Let your knees relax toward the floor, and gently press your elbows down on your knees to increase the stretch. If you are already flexible in this part of your body, grab your toes and lean forward as far as possible while keeping your back straight.

Quadriceps

Lie down on your left side and prop your-self up on your left elbow, as shown. Bend your right leg back and grab your right ankle with your right hand. Gently hold your right ankle and bring your leg back toward your buttocks. Hold the position when you feel a comfortable stretch in the front of your thigh. Release slowly, roll over to your right side, and repeat.

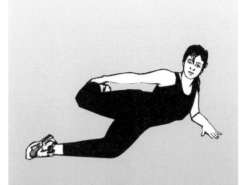

Calves #1

With your hands and feet on the ground, make your body into a V shape. With both feet together, bend your right knee and press your left heel toward the ground, stretching your left calf. Repeat on the other side.

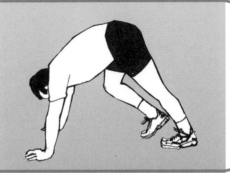

Calves #2

Stand arms-length away from a wall or another solid support. Lean on it with your hands placed shoulder-width apart. Bring your left foot forward, knee bent, while keeping the right leg straight. Lean toward the wall and keep your right heel on the ground while holding the stretch. Switch legs and repeat.

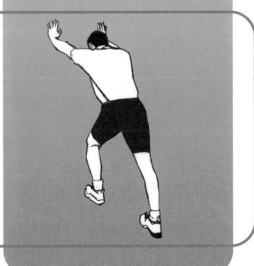

Workload

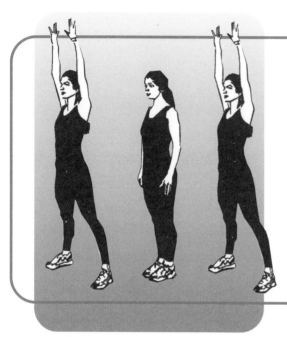

Jumping Jacks

This exercise burns fat and helps improve your hand-eye coordination.

30 to 50 reps

Start with your arms fully extended over-head and your legs apart. While exhaling, simultaneously bring your arms down and touch your hands on each side of the out-side of your thighs while shuffling your feet together, barely lifting them off the ground. Inhale as you return to the starting position and repeat, keeping your arms as straight as possible during the entire movement.

Abdominals/Hips and Legs

These exercises strengthen your core region, and trim and tone your legs.
To be performed on a firm exercise mat.

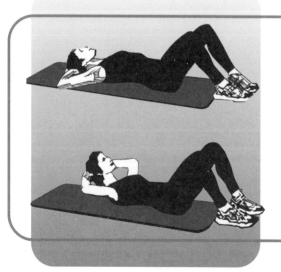

Sit-Ups (Beginner)

20 to 40 reps

Lie on your back with your knees bent, feet flat on the floor with heels up against your mat, and your hands clasped behind your head. Slowly raise your shoulder blades up a few inches while bringing your chest toward your knees. Exhale while curling up. Slowly lower your body to the starting position and repeat.

Sit-Ups *(Intermediate)*

20 to 40 reps

Lie on your back with your knees bent, feet flat on the floor with heels up against your mat, your thumbs clasped with your arms fully extended, as shown. Slowly raise your arms (keeping them straight) toward your knees and perform a full sit-up. Exhale while sitting up. Slowly lower your body to the starting position and repeat.

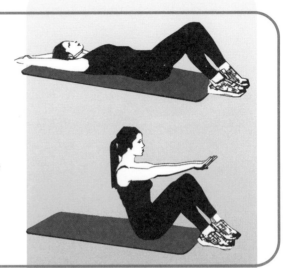

Sit-Ups *(Advanced)*

20 to 40 reps

Lie on your back with your knees bent, feet flat on the floor with heels up against your mat, and your hands on your ears, as shown. Slowly raise your body all the way up, bringing your elbows toward your knees. Exhale while sitting up. Slowly lower your body to the starting position and repeat.

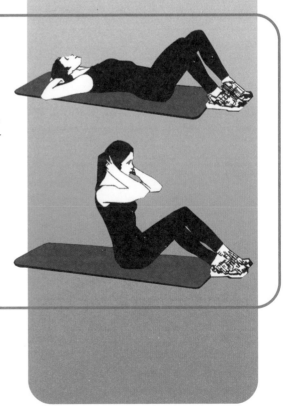

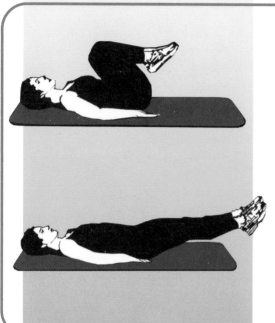

Leg-Outs

**20 reps, rest 30 seconds,
then do another 20 reps**

Lying on your back, with your hands under your buttocks, palms down, bring both knees in toward your chest. Slowly straighten your legs out with toes pointed and repeat. Inhale while bringing your knees toward your chest; exhale as you straighten your legs. Beginners should straighten their legs out at a higher angle. As you get stronger, try to bring your legs lower (about two inches from the ground) while straightening them.

Please note: as your back and abs get stronger, you can move your hands from under your buttocks to behind your neck to intensify the exercise.

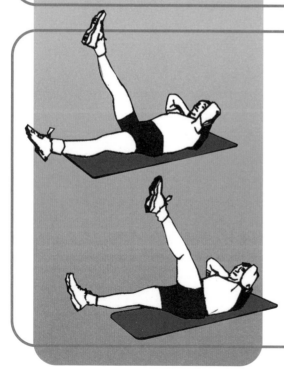

Alternates

**20 reps, rest 30 seconds,
then do another 20 reps**

Lie on your back with your hands under your buttocks, palms down, or clasped behind your neck, as shown, with legs straight and toes pointed. Raise your right leg to a 90-degree angle; your left leg stays on the floor. Pressing the small of your back into the floor, lower your right leg as you simultaneously lift your left leg to a 90-degree angle. Continuously repeat this scissoring motion.

Please note: as your back and abs get stronger, you can move your hands from under your buttocks to behind your neck to intensify the exercise.

Vertical Scissors

20 reps, rest 30 seconds, then do another 20 reps

Lie on your back, hands at your sides or next to or under your buttocks, with palms facing down. Raise both legs to a 90-degree angle. Pressing your back into the floor and with toes pointed and legs straight, slowly open your legs as wide as possible and then bring them back together while exhaling, keeping your toes pointed and your legs straight as you repeat the exercise.

Please note: if you have poor hamstring flexibility, do not attempt this exercise until you have improved that flexibility.

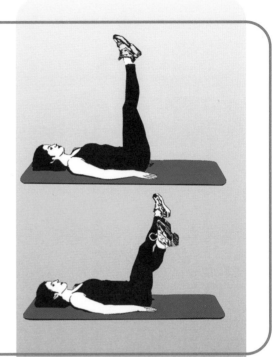

Elbows to Knees

20 reps

Lying on your back, raise your knees and feet toward your chest in a tucked position. Clasp your hands at the base of your neck. Gently curl your upper body, bringing your elbows toward your knees while exhaling. Slowly lower your back and shoulders to the mat while inhaling and repeat. Keep your lower body motionless throughout the entire movement.

Please note: if you cannot touch your elbows to your knees, that's okay. Just reach as far as possible. As you lose weight and increase your hamstring flexibility, you will eventually be able to touch your elbows to your knees.

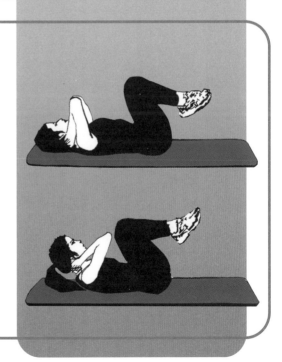

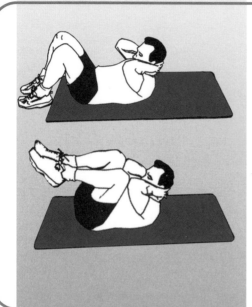

Knees to Elbows

20 reps

Lie on your back with your hands clasped behind the base of your neck. Raise your knees and feet in a tucked position toward your elbows, keeping your lower back pressed against the floor while exhaling. Lower your toes to the ground while inhaling and repeat. Keep the upper half of your body motionless throughout the entire movement.

Please note: if you cannot touch your knees to your elbows, that's okay. Just reach as far as you can. As you lose weight and increase your hamstring flexibility, you will eventually be able to touch your knees to your elbows.

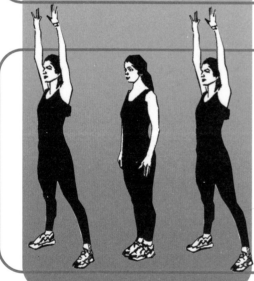

Jumping Jacks

30 to 50 reps

Start with your arms fully extended overhead and your legs apart. While exhaling, simultaneously bring your arms down and touch your hands on each side of the outside of your thighs while shuffling your feet together, barely lifting them off the ground. Inhale as you return to the starting position and repeat, keeping your arms as straight as possible during the entire movement.

Cool-down

Three minutes of easy biking or walking leisurely.

Please note: as you get in better shape, you may borrow additional exercises from the endurance exercise regimens (see chapter 8). Do not, however, do any of the strength exercises until you have shed weight; otherwise, you may bulk up!

Fitness Prescriptions for Endurance

Endurance training mimics how your body functions for golf more than any other form of exercise. To help you further understand this point, *endurance* simply means repetitive movements with a light weight—that is, moving the same weight repetitively without the taking a break. Now, think about your golf swing. If you shoot roughly 85 for a round, and subtract 30 to 35 strokes for putting, you have between 50 and 55 for the number of times you need to swing either a wood or an iron during your golf match. That means you are swinging pretty much the same weight (golf clubs being generally equal in weight even though different in balance) more than 50 times each time you play a round of golf. This is a perfect example of the term functional fitness: in terms of golf, how fit you are for the game. Thinking about the physical requirements of the game will help you determine what type of exercises you should perform to improve your score. How strong, how flexible, how aerobically fit do you truly need to be in order to play golf? I don't believe in doing fewer than 25 reps of any exercise with a light to moderate weight while training for golf (unless you are strength training and are small in size, not overweight, and have a difficult time adding and keeping muscle mass on your frame).

Big muscles are not necessary to hit the golf ball farther. In fact, they can actually hinder your swing unless you have excellent flexibility and range of motion throughout your entire body. Most people don't normally have both, so they can't draw on even half their strength. There is one reason why professional golfers don't look like linebackers. Different sports require different types of training.

What most people don't understand is that gaining strength and endurance is not only accomplished by lifting heavy weights. Remember, your fitness regimen should mimic your sport. When do you ever lift an object more than a few pounds while playing golf? There is a fine line between endurance and strength. You can possess both endurance and strength if you train for endurance, yet it is very hard to possess endurance if you primarily train for strength.

The most effective way to build endurance is to go quickly from exercise to exercise without taking too much time to rest between sets. Your goal is to keep your weight the same until you can perform at least forty to fifty reps per exercise before you increase the resistance and/or weight. The more reps you perform, the stronger you become, and the more reps you perform, the more calories you burn. The more you get your muscles used to moving in a way that will help your golf swing, the more likely it will be that you will eventually add distance, and control, to all your shots.

As you exercise to improve your endurance, you will need to rest a bit, at least initially, between exercises. But you still want to keep moving to get the most out of your workouts. During the exercise regimen outlined here, you will sometimes see the term *active rest*. *Active rest* means that, after immediately finishing one particular exercise, you need your heart rate to come down before you attempt your next exercise because you cannot perform the upcoming exercise with 100 percent efficiency without having to stop at some point to catch your breath. Anaerobic exercises, such as chin-ups or push-ups, shoot your heart rate up, so you will need to recover (rest) a bit before you will be able to go on to your next exercise. Depending on how intense your previous exercise was, you will need to rest, but you don't want to suddenly stop or sit down. Instead, continue to move your body, but in a fashion that allows you to rest between exercises; hence the term active rest. There are a number of ways you can actively rest when needed: you can perform side benders, walk or bike leisurely, or do a combination of both. The key is to keep moving your body in a way that allows your entire system to slow down and recover, enabling you to go onto your next exercise and complete it without taking a break in the middle. As you condition your body and get in better shape, you will need to take fewer rest periods or you will need less time during them. That's when you know you are getting in better physical condition, because your cardiovascular system is working more efficiently.

The term *cross-training* is often used in fitness. For golf, cross-training is essential because it helps reduce potential boredom and overuse trauma. Overuse syndromes or muscular imbalances result from overtraining or performing only one type of cardiovascular activity. For instance, if you run as your main aerobic exercise, you should add another type of exercise, such as biking, jumping rope, or perhaps using an elliptical machine to your routine. Another important benefit of cross-training is that you could be "aerobically fit" to walk but not aerobically fit to run or bike or jump rope. That's because you use different muscle groups at different levels of intensity for each exercise and your system gets used to working in one particular way. So it's important to cross-train in order to become aerobically fit and able to perform a number of cardio and aerobic activities. For example, say you have to walk up a steep incline or hill to get to your next golf shot. The problem is that you are only used to walking on a treadmill without an incline. When you finally get to your ball, you find yourself taxed, and now you need to hit a difficult shot while your entire system is still trying to recover. Nine out of ten times, you will either hit an errant shot or you won't be able to execute your swing with the power needed to get the golf ball toward the green because your system cannot adapt that quickly.

With normal aerobic activity, our bodies work efficiently under constant conditions. When we include interval training, which works on the principle of moving in and out of steady activities, our bodies react differently and the exercise seems harder and more demanding. *Interval training* means exercising at different levels of intensity during a particular activity or exercise. Running and then walking is a good example of interval training. Let's say you run at 7 mph for a short period of time, then you walk to recover, then you step it up again and run when your system allows you to do so. You can also interval-train while performing anaerobic exercise, such as doing sit-ups at a fast pace or in a more advanced position, then doing sit-ups at a slower pace or in an easier body position. Another example is bench-pressing, when you do ten reps at 100 pounds, then eight reps at 80 pounds, then six reps at 60 pounds—that kind of interval work allows you to continue performing the same exercise at different levels of intensity so you can exercise longer.

The benefits of cross-training and interval training also include raising your basal metabolic rate (BMR) and burning more calories during your entire workout regimen. As you increase intensity, you also increase the total number of calories burned, which is important for weight loss or weight maintenance. It also saves you time and shortens your exercise period a bit, because you might need to exercise thirty minutes performing just one type of exercise to equal the calories burned if you were to both cross-train and interval-train. The endurance fitness regimens in this chapter are a combination of cross-training and interval training so that you can maximize your time and reach your goals in a safer and more efficient manner.

Exercising for Endurance

Here are some guidelines to consider as you plan your endurance fitness regimen:

- Work out at least two to three days a week, performing a full body regimen to gain maximum benefits.

- Minimize the amount of time between exercises, and if you need to rest, make sure to take active rests, as opposed to sitting or doing nothing.

- If you are overweight by more than ten pounds, you need to do at least two days of additional aerobic conditioning each week.

- Work on increasing the number of repetitions to a minimum of forty before you add weight or resistance.

- If you are top-heavy, lower the amount of weights for all upper body exercises.

- If you are bottom-heavy, lower the weights/resistance for all lower body exercises.

- If you have a tendency to bulk up both in your upper and lower body, keep the weight/resistance low to moderate for all exercises until you lose some weight. Then you can increase the amount of weight/resistance.

- Your workout time should be split evenly between aerobic and anaerobic exercises in order to achieve the best results.

The exercise prescriptions that follow are designed to be performed at your gym or health club. If you don't belong to a gym or health club, or if you travel often, I have given you substitute exercises so that you can still do them. If you enjoy working out at home, invest in some fitness equipment, specifically a bike or treadmill, a combo chin-dip unit and some weights, and a weighted straight bar and dumbbells. If you are a beginner exerciser, watch the enclosed DVD first so that you'll feel more confident about proper form, alignment, and technique. The DVD is an educational tool to demonstrate how the stretches and exercises should be performed. Please follow the fitness prescriptions outlined here and, when needed, watch the DVD to see how that particular exercise is properly executed.

Fitness Equipment for Endurance Workouts

You want to keep your fitness program as simple as possible, so your exercise equipment should be easy to use. Make sure that you can perform all the exercises no matter where you are because consistency and frequency are the keys to your success!

Although you may use any piece of aerobic fitness equipment for the aerobic portion of your workouts, I highly recommend that you use a recumbent stationary bike. It's easy on your back and knees and it's comfortable, so you'll want to stick with your exercise regimen.

Choose one or more of the following pieces of aerobic equipment: a recumbent or upright stationary bike, a treadmill, an elliptical machine, or a cross-trainer. If you don't have access to any equipment, walk or jog instead.

You may also want:

- A firm exercise mat for abdominal exercises
- A padded bench for upper and lower body exercises
- A chin-up bar and a dip bar for upper body exercises
- A lightweight (2–4-lb.) collapsible aerobic bar for upper body exercises and side benders
- An 8–10-lb. weighted bar for women and a 15–20-lb. weighted bar for men for upper body exercises
- Some 5- and 10-lb. weighted plates to add to the weight bar for lower body exercises
- A beaded or peg jump rope (see page 84 for jump rope instructions)

Your workouts are designed to improve your endurance, help you lose body fat, and tone both your upper and lower body. Please note that if you want to lose some extra weight, do extra aerobic exercise on the days in between structured workouts, and if you want to add some weight or mass, you may borrow some of the exercises from the strength workouts detailed in chapter 9. Remember to keep the weights low to moderate if you are looking to lose some weight.

If you need a break at any time during your exercise regimen, you can get on a stationary bike or any other piece of aerobic equipment or walk for one to three minutes to allow your heart rate to come down safely before you resume. Also, if you want to pay more attention to either your upper body, your midsection, or your lower body, you can perform more repetitions or do an extra set of exercises that target that region.

If you can perform more repetitions with any exercise, please go ahead and do so. If not, keep track of how many repetitions you do for all your exercises and as you increase your fitness level you will be able to comfortably increase the number of repetitions you perform. Try to add two repetitions for each exercise every two weeks, working up to fifty to sixty repetitions for each exercise, and work up to five to ten minutes of continuously jumping rope.

While exercising, if you feel that these workouts are not challenging enough for you, add repetitions and a pound or two to your current weight bar; or tension/resistance to your exercises where applicable; and both speed (revolutions per minute/rpm) and duration to your jump rope segments.

Before you start any fitness plan, consult your healthcare professional or doctor for approval.

Program A: Full Body Exercise Regimen

Frequency: 2 to 3 days a week, every other day.
Duration: 60 to 75 minutes, depending on your current level of fitness.

Warm-up and aerobic segment

Do one of the following for 20 minutes:

- Bike with moderate to high tension/resistance at 80+ rpm or 12+ mph.

- Walk at 4+ mph or jog at 6+ mph with slight hills or incline.

- If you are using an elliptical machine or a cross-trainer, do moderate to high speed with light resistance and/or incline.

Stretch

Hold each of the following stretches for 30 to 60 seconds. To aid you with your stretches and to help you memorize your stretch routine, watch the DVD.

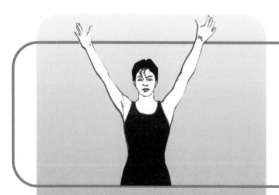

Arm Circles

With arms outstretched, slowly circle your arms backward for five revolutions, and then five revolutions forward. Try to create as big an arc as possible.

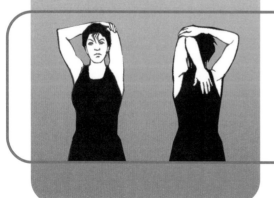

Triceps

With arms overhead, gently pull your left elbow behind your head with your right hand. Hold when you reach a comfortable stretch in the shoulder and upper back. Switch arms and repeat.

Shoulders and Chest

Grasp your hands behind your back, with palms facing each other. Slightly bend your knees and lift your arms up as you bend forward at the waist. Hold when you feel a comfortable stretch in the shoulders and chest.

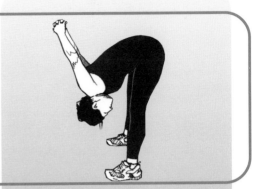

Arms, Upper Back, and Chest

While standing upright, reach behind you with your right arm, keeping it perfectly straight, and grasp onto a door molding or any other immovable object. Now look over your left shoulder and hold the stretch. Switch to your left arm and repeat.

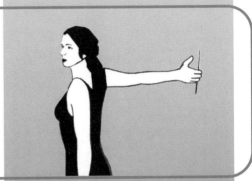

Spinal Twist #1

Sitting on the ground, keep your left leg straight, right arm behind you for support. Cross your right leg over your left knee and place your right foot outside your left knee. With your left hand or elbow on your right knee, slowly twist, and look over your right shoulder while simultaneously pulling your knee in the opposite direction; hold. You will feel pressure in the hip, side, and back. Repeat on the opposite side.

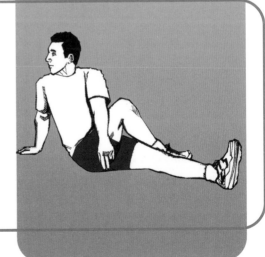

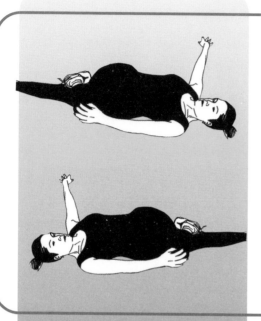

Spinal Twist #2

While lying on your back, bend your right leg, and hook your right toe behind your left knee, as shown. Keep your right arm out straight at a 90-degree angle to maintain your balance. Take your left arm and hand and push down gently on your right knee while keeping your right shoulder blade flat on the ground at all times. Turn your head to look toward your right hand while keeping your head resting on the ground at all times. Keep applying pressure with your left hand and try to get the right knee to touch the ground without the right shoulder blade leaving the ground. Repeat on the other side.

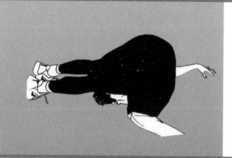

Roll Backs

While lying on your back, roll backward, and balance yourself on your upper shoulders, as shown. Try to extend your legs straight over your forehead and behind you as you hold the stretch.

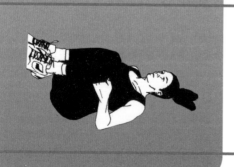

Knees to Chest

While lying on your back, bring both knees up toward your chest, as shown. Grab your right and left legs under your knees with each hand and pull your knees and legs in toward your chest.

Hamstrings—Legs Together

Sit down on the ground with your legs straight, ankles flexed. Bend forward from your hips and reach out toward your toes. Based on your flexibility, grab onto your socks, shoelaces, or toes and hold the stretch. You will feel tension just behind the knees, upper calves, and in the lower back area.

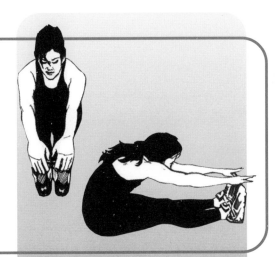

Hamstrings—Legs Apart

Sitting on the ground, with legs straight and apart, bend forward from the hips and reach toward your toes. Based on your flexibility, grab onto your toes or, if this is not possible, your socks or shoelaces.

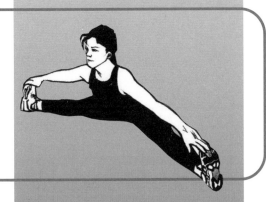

Groin

In a sitting position, pull the soles of your feet together, and grab hold of your ankles. Gently pull your heels toward the groin area. Let your knees relax toward the floor, and gently press your elbows down on your knees to increase the stretch. If you are already flexible in this part of your body, grab your toes and lean forward as far as possible while keeping your back straight.

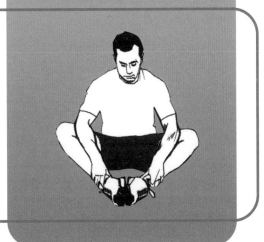

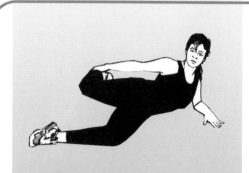

Quadriceps

Lie down on your left side and prop yourself up on your left elbow, as shown. Bend your right leg back and grab your right ankle with your right hand. Gently hold your right ankle and bring your leg back toward your buttocks. Hold the position when you feel a comfortable stretch in the front of your thigh. Release slowly, roll over to your right side, and repeat.

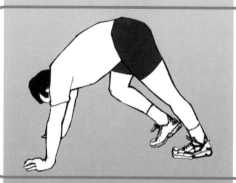

Calves #1

With hands and feet on the ground, make your body into a V shape. With both feet together, bend your right knee and press your left heel toward the ground, stretching your left calf. Repeat on the other side.

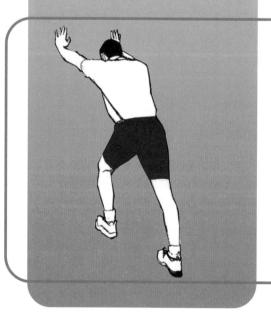

Calves #2

Stand arms-length away from a wall or another solid support. Lean on it with your hands placed shoulder-width apart. Bring your left foot forward, knee bent, while keeping the right leg straight. Lean toward the wall and keep your right heel on the ground while holding the stretch. Switch legs and repeat.

Workload

Upper Body

These exercises work your upper body, forearms, triceps, and biceps. If you don't have access to a chin/dip unit or you cannot perform these exercises, do the exercises described in Option II, on page 128.

Option I:

Chin-Ups

5 to 12 reps, then 40 to 60 side benders to catch your breath

Use the chinning bar about 6 inches higher off the floor than you can reach (if possible) with your arms extended overhead, as shown. Hold the bar with your palms facing you about 6 to 8 inches apart. Pull yourself up, trying to get your chin at or above the bar, and then return to the starting position. Try to keep your back slightly hyperextended and do not swing back and forth; exhale while chinning up and inhale while lowering your body down to the starting position. When you lower yourself back down to the starting position, make sure you fully extend your arms so they are as straight as possible. You may also do this exercise with palms facing away from you (pull-ups).

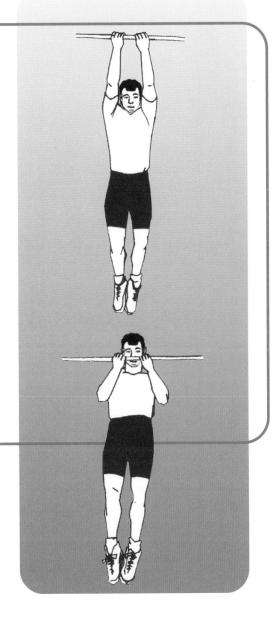

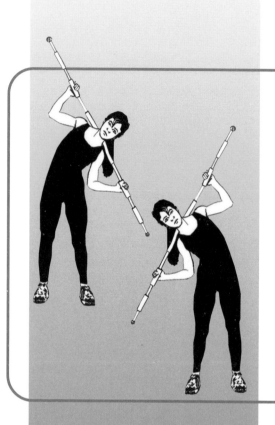

If you need an active rest here, perform 40 to 60 side benders.

Side Benders

While standing upright, legs hip-width apart, place the aerobic bar on your neck, as shown. Bend to the left side as far as possible without moving your hips and legs. Now bend back to the right side as far as possible. Do not stop in the middle. Keep repeating the movement back and forth at a slow pace until you've caught your breath.

Do not use more than a 4-lb. aerobic bar while performing side benders if you are overweight so as not to build too much muscle under the fat. If you are not overweight, you may use up to a 15-lb. weighted bar to perform side benders.

Dips

5 to 12 reps

Hold yourself erect on the bars with your arms straight, as shown. Keeping your elbows pressed into your sides, lower your body by bending your elbows. Continue lowering down until your elbows are bent at a 90-degree angle, then press back to the starting position. Do not let your body swing back and forth. Exhale as you press up and inhale as you lower your body. You may also perform this exercise while facing outwards, with your back facing the back of the dip unit.

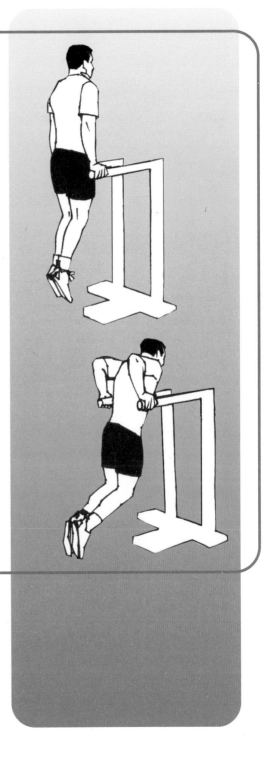

Option II:

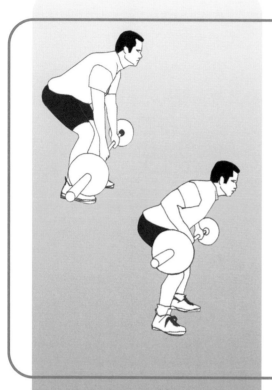

Bent-Over Rows

Use either the standard bar or an Olympic bar with 20–60 lbs. of weight added on.

Two sets of 10 to 15 reps

Place the bar in front of you, your knees slightly bent, your hands wider than shoulder-width apart, and bend over with your torso parallel to the floor. Pull the bar straight up toward the lower part of your chest while exhaling. Keeping your lower body still throughout the entire exercise, lower the bar to the starting position while inhaling, and keep your head up and your back as straight as possible. This can also be done with a narrow grip. Maintain moderate speed throughout the entire movement.

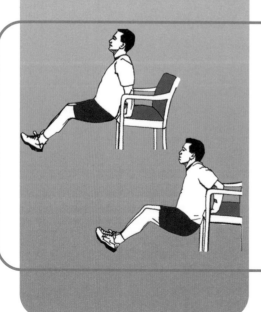

Chair Dips

10 to 20 reps

Position yourself with your arms straight, palms down, holding onto a chair, bench, or a step. Place your weight on your back heels with your knees slightly bent, as shown, and lower your body, trying to touch the ground lightly with your buttocks, and then push yourself up toward the starting position. Exhale as you push up and inhale as you lower your buttocks toward the ground.

Lower Body

These exercises work your quadriceps, hamstrings, and buttocks, and will strengthen your legs to prevent fatigue when walking 18 holes.

Lunges

10 to 20 reps

Place either an aerobic bar, a weighted bar, or a weighted bar with 5–10-lb. plates on each side on the back of your neck across your shoulders, with your hands wider than shoulder-width apart and your feet hip-width apart, as shown. Point your toes straight ahead and step forward with your right leg slightly farther than average stride length, landing right foot heel to toe and coming to a complete stop. Keep your torso erect, inhale, and descend by bending your knees and dropping your hips straight down, stopping short of your left knee touching the ground. While exhaling, push off your right leg and return to the starting position with your feet hip-width apart. Do this exercise one leg at a time and then switch legs and work your left leg.

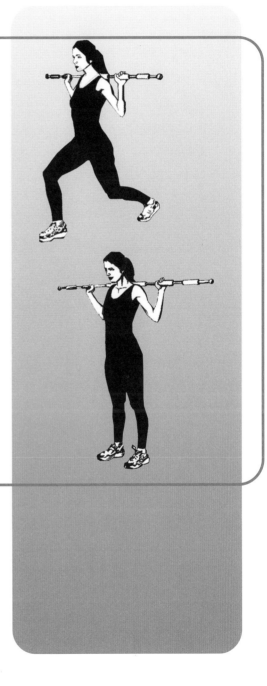

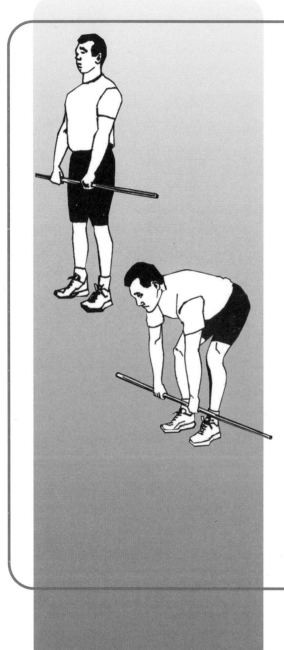

Dead Lifts

Two sets of 15 reps

If you have extremely poor hamstring flexibility or lower back issues, skip this exercise and work your hamstrings instead by performing two additional sets of leg curls (page 199).

Grip either an aerobic bar, a weighted bar, or a weighted bar with 5- to 10-lb. plates on each side with your palms facing your body and about shoulder-width apart. Hold the bar with your arms fully extended in front of your thighs, your elbows at your sides. Your feet can be either close together or wide apart and your knees slightly bent. Keeping the bar close to the front of your thighs, inhale while you slowly bend at the waist toward your toes and go as far down as possible, trying to touch your toes with the bar, keeping your knees slightly bent. While exhaling, bend back up, keeping your arms fully extended throughout the entire exercise. Squeeze your buttocks as you straighten up, and slightly arch your back at the top.

Please note: if you possess great hamstring flexibility and have no back issues, you may do this exercise with your legs straight and/or standing on a step or a bench. Try to go past your toes, touching the ground with the bar.

Step-Ups

Two sets of 15 reps

Stand in front of a bench or step and place either an aerobic bar, a weighted bar, or a weighted bar with 5- to 10-lb. plates on each side on the back of your neck across your shoulders, with your hands wider than shoulder-width apart and your feet hip-width apart, as shown. While keeping your back straight, place your left leg flat on the bench and step up off the ground with your right, while placing all your weight on the left leg and bringing your right leg onto the bench. Lower your right leg to the starting position and repeat. Do this exercise one leg at a time and then switch legs and work your right leg.

As you gain strength and stability, you can step up to a higher bench to increase the intensity.

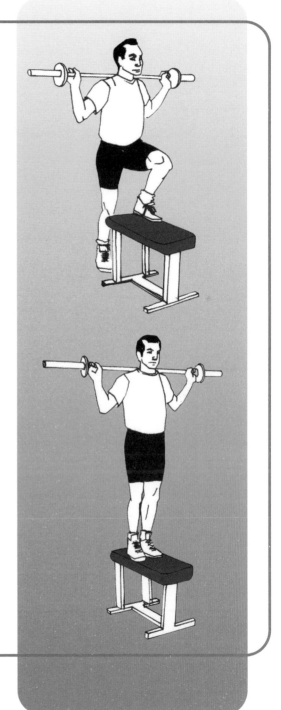

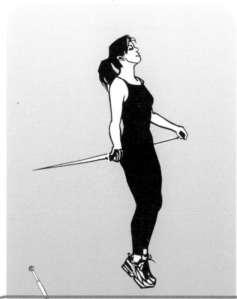

Endurance Segment

Jump rope for 1 minute, then spend 3 minutes biking, walking, jogging, or using any aerobic equipment of your choice—with moderate intensity. If you cannot jump rope, then perform 5 minutes on your choice of aerobic equipment.

Please note: you may also perform side benders after your aerobic segment or at any time during your workout to catch your breath and/or work on your obliques and range of motion.

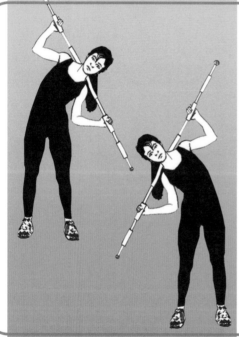

Side Benders

While standing upright, legs hip-width apart, place the aerobic bar on your neck, as shown. Bend to the left side as far as possible without moving your hips or legs. Maintain your stability. Now bend back to the right side as far as possible. Do not stop in the middle. Keep repeating the movement back and forth at a slow pace until you've caught your breath.

To keep from building up too much muscle under the fat, do not use more than a 4-lb. aerobic bar while performing side benders. As you lose weight, increase the weight of the bar as you perform side benders.

Now repeat the exercises for your upper body (Option I, page 125, or Option II, page 128), then repeat the exercises for your lower body (page 129).

Abdominals/Hips and Legs

These exercises strengthen your core and tone your legs.
To be performed on a firm exercise mat.

Sit-Ups *(Intermediate)*

20 to 40 reps

Lie on your back with your knees bent, feet flat on the floor with heels up against your mat, your thumbs clasped with your arms fully extended, as shown. Slowly raise your arms (keeping them straight) toward your knees and perform a full sit-up. Exhale while sitting up. Slowly lower your body to the starting position as you inhale and repeat.

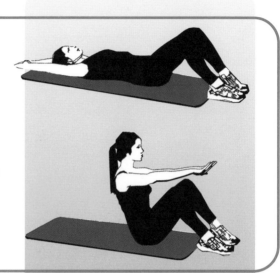

Sit-Ups *(Advanced)*

20 to 40 reps

Lie on your back with your knees bent, feet flat on the floor with heels up against your mat, your hands on your ears, as shown. Slowly raise your body all the way up, bringing your elbows toward your knees. Exhale while sitting up. Slowly lower your body to the starting position and repeat.

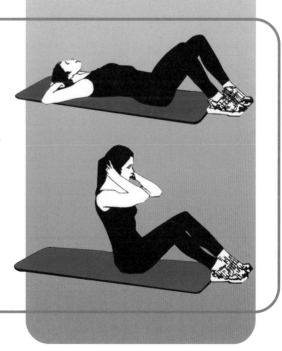

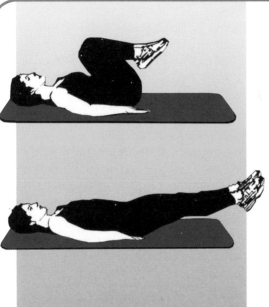

Leg-Outs

20 reps, rest 30 seconds, then do another 20 reps

Lying on your back, with your hands under your buttocks, palms down, bring both knees in toward your chest. Slowly straighten your legs out with toes pointed and repeat. Inhale while bringing your knees toward your chest; exhale as you straighten your legs. Beginners should straighten their legs out at a higher angle. As you get stronger, try to bring your legs lower (about two inches from the ground) while straightening them.

Please note: as your back and abs get stronger, you can move your hands from under your buttocks to behind your neck to intensify the exercise.

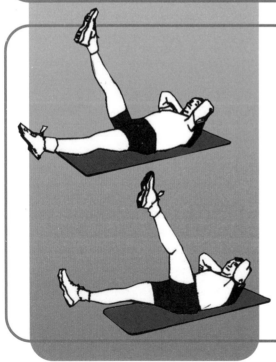

Alternates

20 reps, rest 30 seconds, then do another 20 reps

Lie on your back with your hands under your buttocks, palms down, or clasped behind your neck, as shown, with your legs straight, and toes pointed. Raise your right leg to a 90-degree angle; your left leg stays on the floor. Pressing the small of your back into the floor, lower your right leg as you simultaneously lift your left leg to a 90-degree angle. Continuously repeat this scissoring motion.

Please note: as your back and abs get stronger, you can move your hands from under your buttocks to behind your neck to intensify the exercise.

Vertical Scissors

20 reps, rest 30 seconds,
then do another 20 reps

(Recommended for women only, unless men's inner and outer thighs are weak or need slimming.)

Lie on your back, hands at your sides or next to or under your buttocks, with palms facing down. Raise both legs to a 90-degree angle. Pressing your back into the floor and with toes pointed and legs straight, slowly open your legs as wide as possible and then bring them back together while exhaling, keeping your toes pointed and your legs straight as you repeat.

Please note: if you have poor hamstring flexibility, do not attempt this exercise until you have improved that flexibility. As you get stronger, you can intensify this exercise by extending your arms straight out at a 90-degree angle with palms facing down to help maintain your balance.

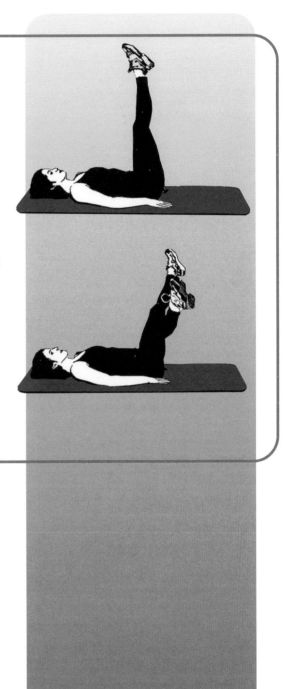

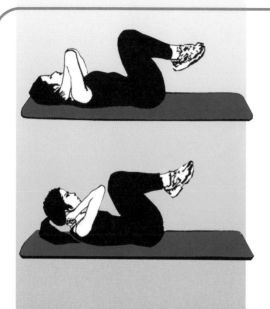

Elbows to Knees

20 reps

Lying on your back, raise your knees and feet toward your chest in a tucked position. Clasp your hands at the base of your neck. Gently curl your upper body, bringing your elbows toward your knees while exhaling. Slowly lower your back and shoulders to the mat while inhaling and repeat. Keep your lower body motionless throughout the entire movement.

Please note: if you cannot touch your elbows to your knees, that's okay. Just reach as far as possible. As you lose weight and increase your hamstring flexibility, you will eventually be able to touch your elbows to your knees.

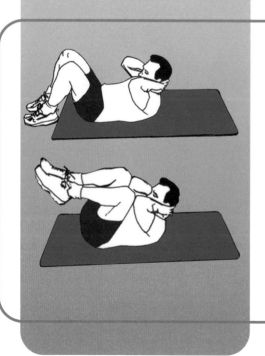

Knees to Elbows

20 reps

Lie on your back with your hands clasped behind the base of your neck. Raise your knees and feet in a tucked position toward your elbows, keeping your lower back pressed against the floor while exhaling. Lower your toes to the ground while inhaling and repeat. Keep the upper half of your body motionless throughout the entire movement.

Please note: if you cannot touch your knees to your elbows, that's okay. Just reach as far as you can. As you lose weight and increase your hamstring flexibility, you will eventually be able to touch your knees to your elbows.

Endurance Segment

Jump rope for 1 to 2 minutes fast, then spend 3 minutes biking, walking, jogging, or using any aerobic equipment of your choice—with moderate intensity. If you cannot jump rope, then perform 5 minutes on your choice of aerobic equipment.

Please note: you may also perform side benders after your aerobic segment or at any time during your workout to catch your breath and/or work on your obliques and range of motion.

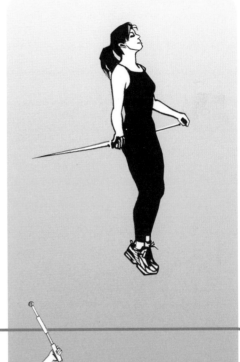

Side Benders

While standing upright, legs hip-width apart, place the aerobic bar on your neck, as shown. Bend to the left side as far as possible without moving your hips or legs. Maintain your stability. Now bend back to the right side as far as possible. Do not stop in the middle. Keep repeating the movement back and forth at a slow pace until you've caught your breath.

To keep from building up too much muscle under the fat, do not use more than a 4-lb. aerobic bar while performing side benders. As you lose weight, increase the weight of the bar as you perform side benders.

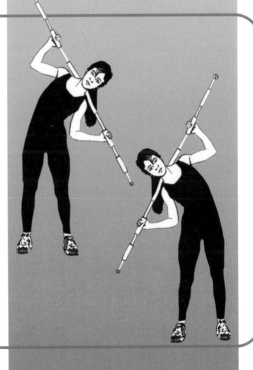

Upper Body
This exercise works your upper back, chest, and arms.

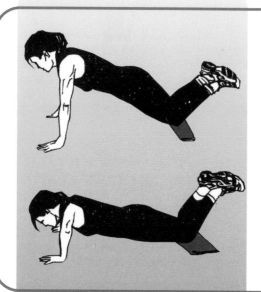

Push-Ups *(Basic)*
Two sets of 15 to 25 reps

On your hands and knees with your ankles crossed, place your knees on a mat or towel with your hands slightly wider than shoulder-width apart, your arms straight, fingers facing forward, and abdominals contracted. While inhaling, lower your chest toward the floor, touching the floor, and then, while exhaling, push up to the starting position. Keep your back straight throughout the entire exercise and repeat. Keep your lower body still through the entire movement.

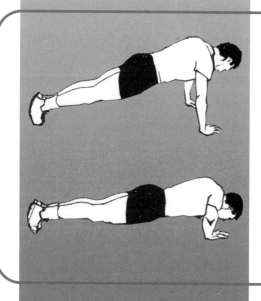

Push-Ups *(Advanced)*
Two sets of 15 to 25 reps

Extend your body on your hands and toes, with your arms straight, and place your hands farther than shoulder-width apart, your fingers facing forward and your abdominals contracted. While inhaling, lower your body toward the floor and lightly touch your chest to the floor. Exhale while pushing up to the starting position and repeat. Do not arch your back or jerk your body during the entire movement.

Endurance Segment

Jump rope for 1 to 2 minutes fast, then spend 3 minutes biking, walking, jogging, or using any aerobic equipment of your choice—with moderate intensity. If you cannot jump rope, then perform 5 minutes on your choice of aerobic equipment.

Please note: you may also perform side benders after your aerobic segment or at any time during your workout to catch your breath and/or work on your obliques and range of motion.

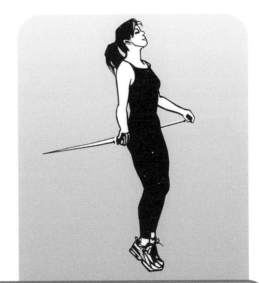

Side Benders

While standing upright, legs hip-width apart, place the aerobic bar on your neck, as shown. Bend to the left side as far as possible without moving your hips or legs. Maintain your stability. Now bend back to the right side as far as possible. Do not stop in the middle. Keep repeating the movement back and forth at a slow pace until you've caught your breath.

To keep from building up too much muscle under the fat, do not use more than a 4-lb. aerobic bar while performing side benders. As you lose weight, increase the weight of the bar as you perform side benders.

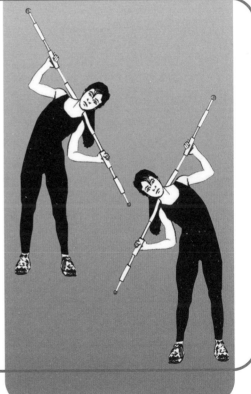

Cool-down

Three minutes of easy biking or walking leisurely.

Program B: Aerobic and Assorted Exercises

Frequency: 2 days a week.

Duration: 50 minutes.

Please note: you should not perform two program As or two program Bs in a row. You should do program A then program B, then A, then B, and so on. Strive to complete two program As and two program Bs each week for maximum results. Also, if you want to rest or need a day off, skip program B, not program A, whenever possible.

Warm-up and aerobic segment

Do one of the following for 30 minutes:

- Bike with moderate to high tension/resistance at 80+ rpm or 12+ mph.
- Walk at 4+ mph or jog at 6+ mph with slight hills or incline.
- If you are using an elliptical machine or a cross-trainer, do moderate to high speed with moderate to high resistance and/or incline.

Stretch

Hold each stretch for 30 to 60 seconds. To aid you with your stretches and to help you memorize your stretch routine, watch the DVD.

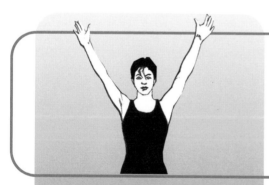

Arm Circles

With arms outstretched, slowly circle your arms backward for five revolutions, and then five revolutions forward. Try to create as big an arc as possible.

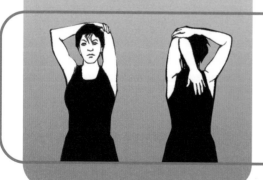

Triceps

With arms overhead, gently pull your left elbow behind your head with your right hand. Hold when you reach a comfortable stretch in the shoulder and upper back. Switch arms and repeat.

Shoulders and Chest

Grasp your hands behind your back, with palms facing each other. Slightly bend your knees and lift your arms up as you bend forward at the waist. Hold when you feel a comfortable stretch in the shoulders and chest.

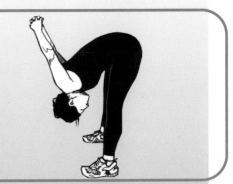

Arms, Upper Back, and Chest

While standing upright, reach behind you with your right arm, keeping it perfectly straight, and grasp onto a door molding or any other immovable object. Now look over your left shoulder and hold the stretch. Switch to your left arm and repeat.

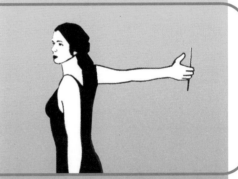

Spinal Twist #1

Sitting on the ground, keep your left leg straight, right arm behind you for support. Cross your right leg over your left knee and place your right foot outside your left knee. With your left hand or elbow on your right knee, slowly twist, and look over your right shoulder while simultaneously pulling your knee in the opposite direction; hold. You will feel pressure in the hip, side, and back. Repeat on the opposite side.

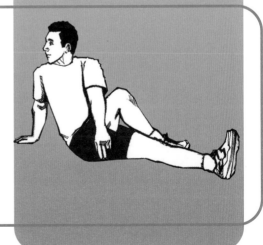

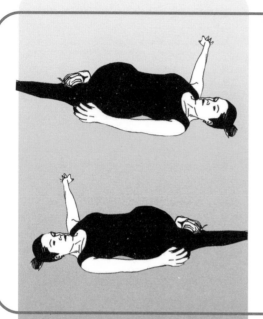

Spinal Twist #2

While lying on your back, bend your right leg, and hook your right toe behind your left knee, as shown. Keep your right arm out straight at a 90-degree angle to balance yourself. Take your left arm and hand and push down gently on your right knee while keeping your right shoulder blade flat on the ground at all times. Turn your head to look toward your right hand while keeping your head resting on the ground at all times. Keep applying pressure with your left hand and try to get the right knee to touch the ground without the right shoulder blade leaving the ground. Repeat on the other side.

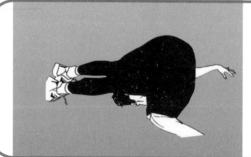

Roll Backs

While lying on your back, roll backward, and balance yourself on your upper shoulders, as shown. Try to extend your legs straight over your forehead and behind you as you hold the stretch.

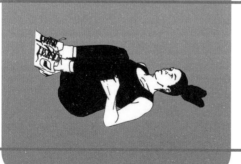

Knees to Chest

While lying on your back, bring both knees up toward your chest, as shown. Grab your right and left legs under your knees with each hand and pull your knees and legs in toward your chest.

Hamstrings—Legs Together

Sit down on the ground with your legs straight, ankles flexed. Bend forward from your hips and reach out toward your toes. Based on your flexibility, grab onto your socks, shoelaces, or toes and hold the stretch. You will feel tension just behind the knees, upper calves, and in the lower back area.

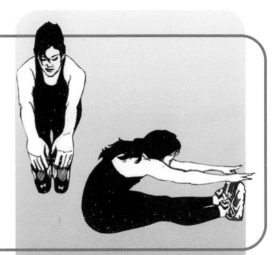

Hamstrings—Legs Apart

Sitting on the ground, with legs straight and apart, bend forward from the hips and reach toward your toes. Based on your flexibility, grab onto your toes or, if this is not possible, your socks or shoelaces.

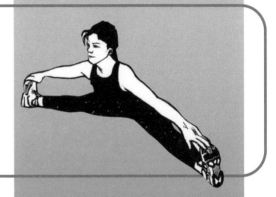

Groin

In a sitting position, pull the soles of your feet together, and grab hold of your ankles. Gently pull your heels toward the groin area. Let your knees relax toward the floor, and gently press your elbows down on your knees to increase the stretch. If you are already flexible in this region of your body, grab your toes and lean forward as far as possible while keeping your back straight.

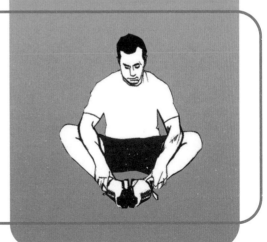

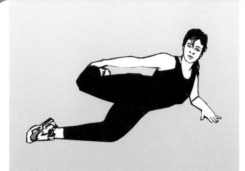

Quadriceps

Lie down on your left side and prop your-self up on your left elbow, as shown. Bend your right leg back and grab your right ankle with your right hand. Gently hold your right ankle and bring your leg back toward your buttocks. Hold the position when you feel a comfortable stretch in the front of your thigh. Release slowly, roll over to your right

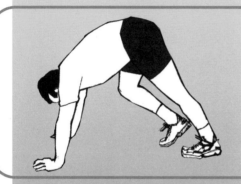

Calves #1

With hands and feet on the ground, make your body into a V shape. With both feet together, bend your right knee and press your left heel toward the ground, stretching your left calf. Repeat on the other side.

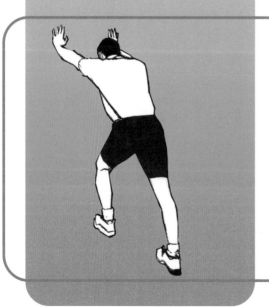

Calves #2

Stand arms-length away from a wall or another solid support. Lean on it with your hands placed shoulder-width apart. Bring your left foot forward, knee bent, while keeping the right leg straight. Lean toward the wall and keep your right heel on the ground while holding the stretch. Switch legs and repeat.

Workload

Endurance Segment

This exercise improves both your aerobic and your anaerobic conditioning.

Squat Thrusts

10 to 20 reps

Stand with your back straight, your feet together or slightly apart. Bend your knees approximately 75 degrees into a squat position, keeping your thighs parallel with the floor, and place your palms down about 8 to 12 inches in front of your toes and slightly wider than shoulder-width apart. Exhaling, kick both legs out behind you, landing with your toes on the floor and your legs straight and fully extended, as shown. Thrust back to a squat position, then stand up with your back straight as you inhale.

To intensify this exercise, you can also do a push-up before you bring in your legs and stand up.

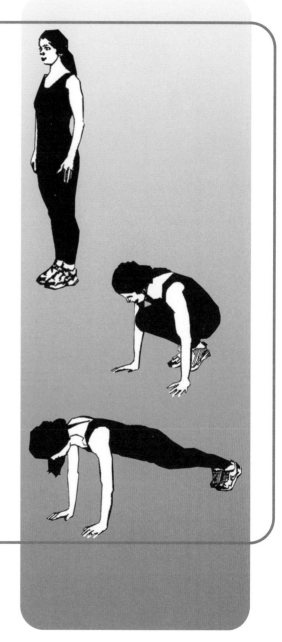

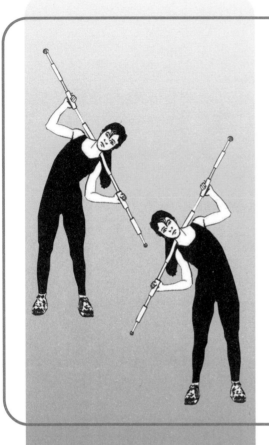

Side Benders

While standing upright, place the aerobic bar on your neck, legs hip-width apart, as shown. Bend to the left side as far as possible without moving your hips or legs. Now bend back to the right side as far as possible. Do not stop in the middle. Keep repeating the movement back and forth at a slow pace until you've caught your breath.

Do not use more than a 4-lb. aerobic bar while performing side benders if you are overweight so as not to build too much muscle under the fat. If you are not overweight, you may use up to a 15-lb. weighted bar to perform side benders.

Upper Body

These exercises work the upper back, chest, and arms. Use an 8–10-lb. weighted bar for women and a 15–20-lb. weighted bar for men.

Push-Outs

20 to 30 reps

Keep your back straight, knees slightly bent, and your feet just wider than hip-width apart. Grip the bar, palms facing down, just wider than shoulder width. Raise the bar up just above your chest line with your elbows up and your wrists firm. Extend your arms straight out, holding the bar level above your chest and exhale. While inhaling, let your arms drop down to the front of your thighs, keeping your arms straight. Bring the bar back to starting position and repeat. Keep your lower body aligned and still throughout the entire exercise. Maintain a moderate speed throughout the movement.

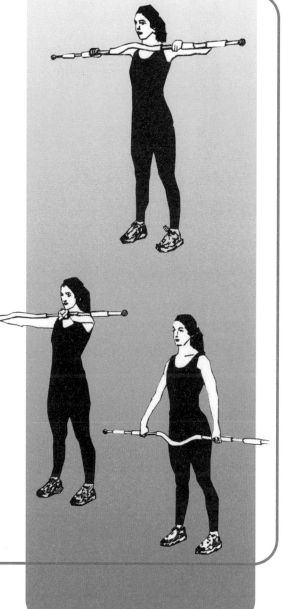

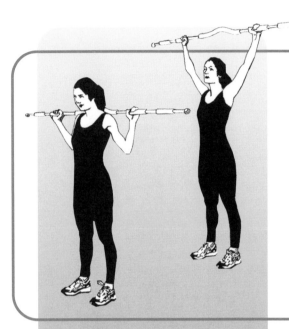

Behind-Neck Press

30 to 40 reps

Grip the bar slightly wider than shoulder width and place it behind your neck and shoulders. Keep your back straight, knees slightly bent, and your feet just wider than hip-width apart. Fully extend your arms upward and raise the bar straight up behind your neck while exhaling. Bend your arms and slowly return the bar to the back of your neck while inhaling and repeat. Make sure you keep the bar as close as possible to the back of your head to avoid neck strain.

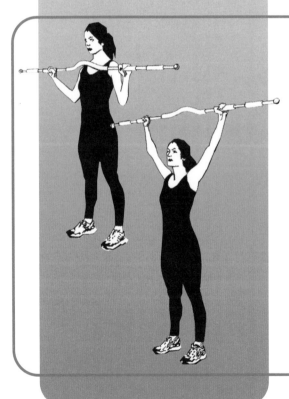

Front Press

30 to 40 reps

Keep your back straight, knees slightly bent, and feet hip-width apart. Grip the bar just past shoulder width and rest the bar across the top of your chest. Fully extend your arms upward and raise the bar straight up while exhaling. Bend your arms and slowly return the bar to the top of your chest while inhaling and repeat. Maintain a moderate speed throughout the entire movement.

Bent-Over Rows

30 to 40 reps

Place the bar on the ground in front of you, knees slightly bent and hands wider than shoulder-width apart, and bend over with your torso parallel to the floor. Pull the bar straight up toward the lower part of your chest while exhaling. Keeping your lower body still throughout the entire exercise, lower the bar to the starting position while inhaling. Keep your head aligned with your back as much as possible. This can also be done with a narrow grip. Maintain a moderate speed throughout the entire movement.

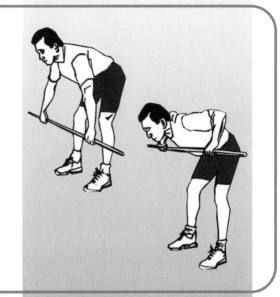

Upright Rows

35 to 45 reps

Keep your back straight, knees slightly bent, and feet hip-width apart. Grip the bar, palms facing down, 6 to 8 inches apart. Hold the bar with your arms fully extended at the front of your thighs. Slowly raise the bar up to your chin, keeping your elbows at or above bar level while exhaling. Return to the starting position while inhaling and repeat. You can also perform this exercise with a wide grip. Maintain a moderate speed throughout the entire movement.

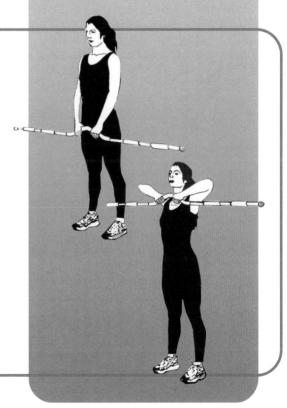

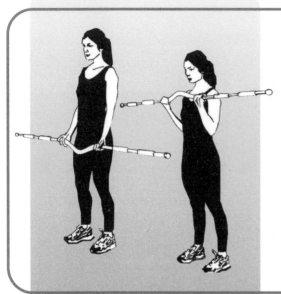

Curls

35 to 45 reps

Keep your back straight, knees slightly bent, and feet hip-width apart. Grip the bar, palms facing up, and shoulder-width apart. Hold the bar with your arms fully extended at the front of your thighs. Keeping your elbows stationary and your wrists firm, curl the bar up to your chest while exhaling. Slowly extend your arms and return the bar to the starting position while inhaling and repeat. This exercise can be done with either a narrow or a wide grip. Maintain a moderate speed throughout the entire movement

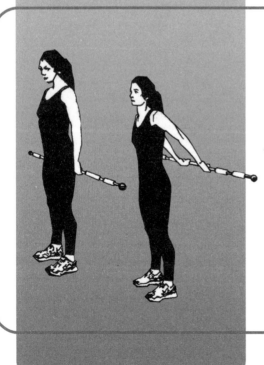

Kick-Backs

20 to 30 reps

Keep your back straight, knees slightly bent, and feet hip-width apart. Grip the bar with arms fully extended at the buttocks, palms facing outward about shoulder-width apart. Keeping your elbows stationary and your wrists firm, lift the bar away from your buttocks as far as possible while exhaling. Keeping your arms straight, lower the bar to your buttocks while inhaling and repeat. Maintain a moderate speed throughout the entire movement.

Advanced Kick-Backs

10 to 20 reps

Keep your back straight, knees slightly bent, and feet hip-width apart. Grip the bar with your arms fully extended at the buttocks, palms facing outward, about shoulder-width apart. Keeping your wrists firm, bend your elbows while lifting the bar up to your lower back and then lift the bar away from your buttocks as far as possible while exhaling. Keeping your arms straight, lower the bar to the buttocks while inhaling and repeat. Maintain a moderate speed throughout the entire movement.

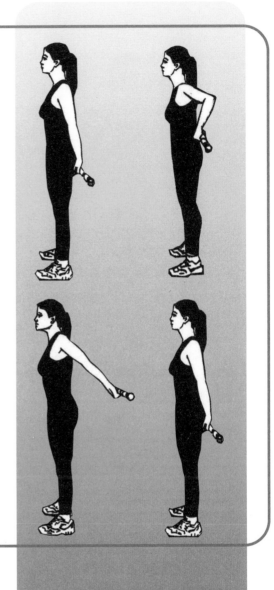

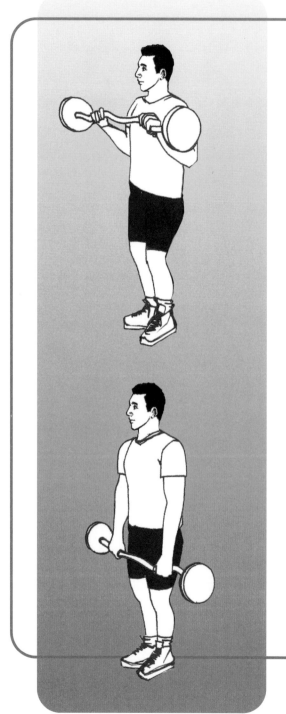

Reverse Curls

20 to 30 reps

Stand up straight, with your knees slightly bent and your feet approximately 12 inches apart. Hold the bar with your palms down about 12 inches apart, your arms fully extended and straight, allowing the bar to rest against the front of your thighs, as shown. Curl the bar up toward your chest as you exhale, keeping your back straight. Don't sway. Keep your elbows as close as possible to your sides as you curl up. Inhaling, return the bar to the starting position and repeat. You may also perform this exercise with a narrow or wide grip.

Abs and Legs

These exercises work your lower abdominal region, your obliques, and your upper thighs.

Leg Lifts

20 to 30 reps, rest 30 seconds,
then do another 10 to 20 reps

Lie on your back on the mat with your body fully extended, your hands palms down under or next to your buttocks, as shown, with your feet 3 to 8 inches from the ground. Keeping your legs straight and your knees locked, raise your legs as high as possible to a 90-degree angle. Lower your legs, keeping them as straight as possible, to the starting position, as shown, and repeat. Exhale as you bring your legs up and inhale as you lower them toward the floor. Focus on keeping your back straight throughout the entire movement—do not arch your back. You may also perform leg lifts with your hands behind your neck and/or off a slant board or bench to make the exercise more intense.

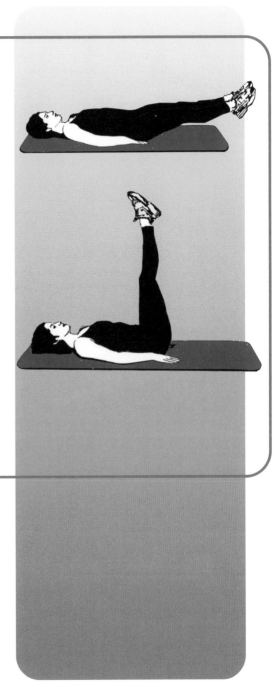

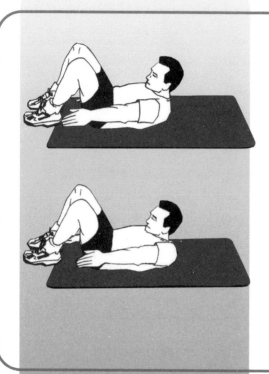

Hand-to-Heel Alternates

30 to 50 reps, rest 30 seconds,
and then do another 20 to 40 reps

Lie on your back with your heels flat up
against an exercise mat, your feet 8 to 12
inches apart, as shown. Raise your shoulders
slightly off the mat and keep your chin
tucked in, as shown. Shift your torso to the
left while keeping your lower body as still
as possible. Reach with your left fingertips
and touch the outside of your left heel.
Then, shift back toward your right heel with
your right fingertips touching the outside
of your right heel, as shown. Do not stop
in the middle as you shift back and forth,
keeping your shoulder blades off the
ground during the entire movement.

Repeat the Endurance Segment

This exercise improves both your aerobic and your anaerobic conditioning.

Squat Thrusts

10 to 20 reps

Stand with your back straight, your feet together or slightly apart. Bend your knees approximately 75 degrees into a squat position, keeping your thighs parallel with the floor, and place your palms down about 8 to 12 inches in front of your toes and slightly wider than shoulder-width apart. Exhaling, kick both legs out behind you, landing with your toes on the floor and legs fully straight and extended, as shown. Thrust back to a squat position, then stand up with your back straight as you inhale.

To intensify this exercise, you can also do a push-up before you bring in your legs and stand up.

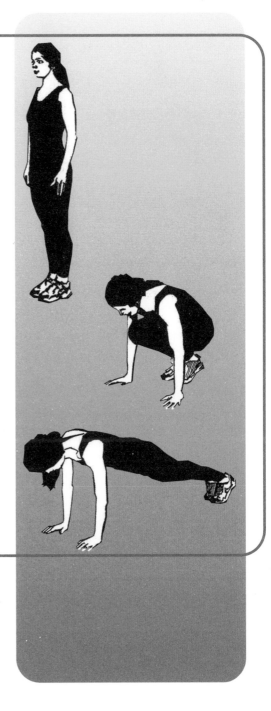

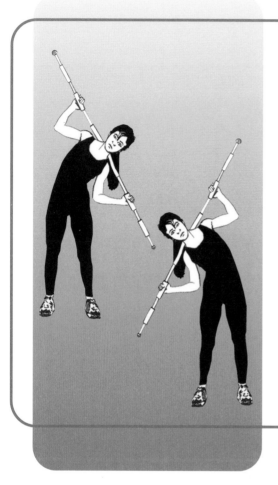

Side Benders

While standing upright, place the aerobic bar on your neck, legs hip-width apart, as shown. Bend to the left side as far as possible without moving your hips or legs. Now bend back to the right side as far as possible. Do not stop in the middle. Keep repeating the movement back and forth at a slow pace until you've caught your breath.

Do not use more than a 4-lb. aerobic bar while performing side benders if you are overweight so as not to build too much muscle under the fat. If you are not overweight, you may use up to a 15-lb. weighted bar to perform side benders.

Cool-down

Three minutes of easy biking or walking leisurely.

Please note: as you progress with your endurance program, try to keep increasing the intensity of each exercise by adding reps, and as you get in better shape, take fewer breaks. In time, you will flow from exercise to exercise without needing rest breaks. This way, you will burn more calories every time you work out.

Fitness Prescriptions for Strengthening Your Body

We all want to be stronger and more fit so we can hit the golf ball with more power and distance. But, because of all the factors involved in strength building, it's more difficult to acquire and build strength than it is to exercise to lose weight or to improve endurance. With strength training, nutrition becomes more important because you need to fuel your body properly for the demands that will be placed on it. If you are looking to gain a considerable amount of muscle mass and/or add weight to your frame, you need to eat a lot, and often, for maximum results. You also need a good night's sleep because of the stress you will be putting on your muscles and joints.

Remember, this chapter is reserved for those who want to add strength and muscle mass to their bodies, so if you're overweight by more than ten to fifteen pounds, I highly recommend that you first lose weight by exercising for weight loss (chapter 7) or slim down by following the workout regimens

for endurance (chapter 8). With strength training, you also need to have access to more fitness equipment than you do with the other workout regimens, and your risk of injury is higher, so you must pay greater attention to form and technique. The fitness equipment needed for strength training is a bit more complicated, so there is a learning curve involved in familiarizing yourself with the various weight machines.

The benefits of strength training are numerous. It will help increase the distance of all your golf shots and improve your overall golf game. Specifically, strength training improves your tone, definition, sports performance, and resistance to injury. Equally important, as we age, our fast-twitch, or explosive, muscle fibers atrophy (deteriorate) at a faster rate than our slow-twitch, or endurance, fibers. Strength training helps to maintain both fiber size and tone, keeping us fit and strong as we age. Strength training, also known as resistance training, improves your strength, which has both physiological and neurological benefits. The physiological changes include hypertrophy (increase in muscle size, the opposite of *atrophy*). The neurological changes include improved coordination.

We often hear the terms *tone* and *definition* in relation to our bodies. Tone is dependent on definition, as the muscles become more aesthetically shaped through work (exercise). Tone is the muscular state in which the muscle has greater than average definition and the fat layer over the muscle is small enough to let that definition show. That's why some overweight individuals who lift heavy amounts of weight don't look toned; they have not shed enough fat to get the desired appearance. Genetically, we all bulk up and add muscle mass at various rates, and, typically, those who are slight in frame or not overweight seem to benefit the most from heavy strength training—aesthetically, at least.

Strength training can be divided into three categories: muscular endurance (chapter 8), muscular strength, and muscular power. The way you choose to exercise is based on your desired strength goal. Strength qualities can be further divided into pure strength or functional strength capabilities. *Pure strength* refers to strength developed outside of a sport or application context, such as weight training. *Functional strength* refers to strength that has been or needs to be developed or transferred to a sport or application context. Leg strength in football is an example of

Exercising properly will make you feel better and give you more energy

functional strength. There is not a lot of research on the relationship between these two qualities, but it is commonly believed in the fitness field that you should build pure strength first, then adapt that strength to your functional sport, such as golf. A good illustration of this would be for golfers to work out via resistance/weight training during the off-season, and then gradually begin to adapt that strength to golf by hitting golf balls and playing rounds. Golfers don't need to lift very heavy weights because they will rarely, if ever, need that type of strength for golf. The term *heavy* in this context refers not only to the amount of weight you are moving, but also how many pounds you are moving compared to your current weight. So, if you are a woman who is 5 feet 9 inches tall and weighs 165 pounds, you don't need to be bench-pressing your weight in order to gain enough strength to hit the golf ball farther.

Is gaining or having more strength a guarantee that you will hit the golf ball farther? Yes, but with a caveat. There is some research comparing golfers who have strength-trained alone versus those who have both strength-trained and done flexibility training. Although both groups showed similar gains in overall body strength, the group that stretched as well had an almost three-times-greater club speed than the group that strength-trained without flexibility training. Although not scientifically measured, the reason the group that stretched had more club speed is most likely due to the increase in range of motion.

To swing a golf club successfully, you need what's called *immediate energy* (muscular stores of energy sufficient for only about one second of maximal effort). Golf requires more immediate energy than almost any other sport—tennis is second, basketball third, and then swimming or running 200 meters. It follows, then, that for golf, repeated work bouts lasting thirty seconds or so are recommended to train and improve the capacity of the immediate energy system. It is also recommended that you do one to three sets of ten to twelve repetitions for each exercise. However, for people who are slight in frame or who are weak, I recommend only small numbers of reps. For people who are already somewhat strong or are overweight, I also recommend a slightly lighter weight because more than that will add too much bulk to your body and could actually hinder your golf swing. Nearly 75 percent or more of a golfer's swing is about utilizing the torso and lower body. Lower body strength is critical for improving overall balance, which is vital to completing a golf swing.

Is it better to train with free weights or weight machines? Although the benefits of free weights/dumbbells outweigh those of weight machines, both are sufficient for helping your golf game. Here's the rule I'd like you to follow: if you are orthopedically sound, have good balance, and don't need a spotter for most exercises, do most of your exercises using free weights. On the other hand, if you have orthopedic concerns, possess poor balance, or don't feel comfortable or confident that you can perform most exercises without someone spotting you, then do most of your exercises using weight machines. As you gain more strength, balance, and confidence, you can eventually switch over to using more free weights.

Exercising to Strengthen Your Body

Here are some guidelines to consider as you plan your strength training fitness regimen:

- Work out at least three days a week, performing a full body regimen to gain the maximum benefit.

- Perform ten to twelve reps with a heavier weight if you are looking to gain mass and size, and fifteen to twenty reps with a lighter weight if you are looking to just gain strength.

- For all aerobic work, keep the resistance/tension high at all times.

- Be sure to stretch before each workout to lower your risk of injury and to increase your range of motion.

- If you feel pain while performing any exercise, stop immediately and do not continue.

- If you experience extreme soreness from your workouts, take an extra day off to recuperate until your body builds up strength and you can recover faster.

- If you want to shed some unwanted weight or fat, do aerobic exercise for one to two additional days a week.

- If your goal is to add mass and weight, do not exercise more than three to four days a week and make sure that at least 75 percent of your workout is anaerobic.

- Do not add weight to an exercise until you can comfortably complete at least twelve repetitions.

- Do not play a round of golf after you perform your strength workout until you have been exercising for a while, so your muscles can get used to the additional demands.

- Make sure to get a good night's sleep and eat nutritiously on the days you workout.

- Make sure you use proper form and body alignment for all exercises. Don't "cheat" and compromise good form for badly executed reps.

The exercise prescriptions that follow are designed to be performed at your gym or health club. If you don't belong to a gym or health club, if you travel often, or if you have the space at home, you may want to buy some home-fitness equipment. If you are a beginner exerciser or are not that knowledgeable about fitness, watch the enclosed DVD so you'll feel more confident about proper form, alignment, and technique. The DVD demonstrates how the stretches and exercises should be performed. Please follow the fitness prescriptions outlined here and, when needed, watch the DVD to see how that particular exercise movement is properly executed.

Fitness Equipment for Strength Training

Choose one or more of the following pieces of aerobic equipment: a recumbent or upright stationary bike, a treadmill, an elliptical machine, a cross-trainer, or, if you don't have access to any equipment, walk or jog instead.
    You will also need:

- A firm exercise mat for abdominal exercises

- A padded incline bench for upper and lower body exercises

- A chin-up bar and dip bar for upper body exercises

- An Olympic bar,* bench, and 200–300 lbs. of weights

- Dumbbells ranging from 10 to 60 lbs.

- A lat pull-down machine for upper body exercises

- A leg extension and leg curl machine for lower body exercises

- A seated leg-press machine for lower body exercises

- A Smith machine (a piece of fitness equipment used to help balance weights on a bar suspended by cables) for lower body exercises

- A lightweight (2–4-lb.) collapsible aerobic bar for calisthenics and side benders

- A 15-lb. weighted straight or curl barbell bar for upper and lower body exercises

- 20–50 lbs. of standard weights to add onto a 15-lb. straight bar for upper and lower body exercises

- A beaded or peg jump rope (see page 84 for jump rope instructions)

*The difference between standard and Olympic bars and weights is that standard bars are shorter and smaller, and the weights have smaller holes, approximately 1 inch in diameter. Olympic bars are longer, larger, and thicker, and are used to hold heavier weights. If you are going to lift more than 75 pounds, use the Olympic weights because they are sturdier and stronger.

If you need a break at any time during your exercise regimen, you can get on a stationary bike or any other piece of aerobic equipment, or walk for one minute, or perform side benders to allow your heart rate to come down safely before you resume. Also, if you want to pay more attention to either your upper body, your midsection, or your lower body, you can perform more repetitions or do an extra set of exercises that target that region.

If you can perform any exercise with more weight than is given in the prescriptions in this chapter, please go ahead and do so. If not, keep track of how many repetitions you do for all of your exercises, and as you increase your fitness level you will then be able to comfortably increase the number of repetitions you perform. Try to add five pounds to each exercise every four weeks. With all of your nonweight exercises and

calisthenics, try to work up to fifty to sixty repetitions and strive for ten minutes of continuous jumping rope.

There are two full body exercise regimens outlined here. Ideally, you should perform program A, rest a day, then perform program B, rest a day, then go back to program A and repeat the sequence. If you skip a workout day or need an extra rest day, you may resume with either workout. Do not perform program A and program B on back-to-back days unless you are a finely tuned athlete. If you want to exercise on the days in between, do some aerobic exercise, stretching, and abdominal exercises only.

Please note: if you are trying to add weight and/or mass, do not do aerobic exercise on days in between programs.

Before you start any fitness plan, consult your healthcare professional or doctor for approval.

Program A: Full Body Exercise Regimen

Frequency: 2 days a week.
Duration: 60 to 75 minutes, depending on your current level of fitness.

Warm-up and aerobic segment

Do one of the following for 12 minutes:

- Bike with high tension/resistance at 70+ rpm or 12+ mph.

- Walk at 4+ mph or jog at 6+ mph with extreme hills or incline.

- If you are using an elliptical machine or a cross-trainer, do moderate speed with high resistance and/or incline.

Stretch

Hold each of the following stretches for 30 to 60 seconds. To aid you with your stretches and to help you memorize your stretch routine, watch the DVD.

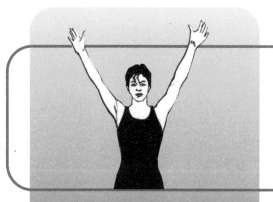

Arm Circles

With arms outstretched, slowly circle your arms backward for five revolutions, and then five revolutions forward. Try to create as big an arc as possible.

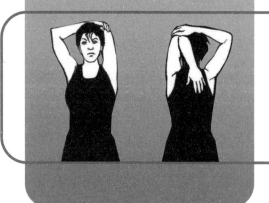

Triceps

With arms overhead, gently pull your left elbow behind your head with your right hand. Hold when you reach a comfortable stretch in the shoulder and upper back. Switch arms and repeat.

Shoulders and Chest

Grasp your hands behind your back, with palms facing each other. Slightly bend your knees and lift your arms up as you bend forward at the waist. Hold when you feel a comfortable stretch in the shoulders and chest.

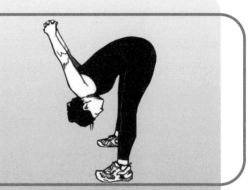

Arms, Upper Back, and Chest

While standing upright, reach behind you with your right arm, keeping it perfectly straight, and grasp onto a door molding or any other immovable object. Now look over your left shoulder and hold the stretch. Switch to your left arm and repeat.

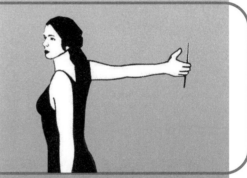

Spinal Twist #1

Sitting on the ground, keep your left leg straight, right arm behind you for support. Cross your right leg over your left knee and place your right foot outside your left knee. With your left hand or elbow on your right knee, slowly twist, and look over your right shoulder while simultaneously pulling your knee in the opposite direction; hold. You will feel pressure in the hip, side, and back. Repeat on the opposite side.

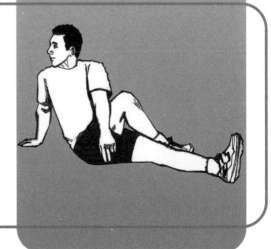

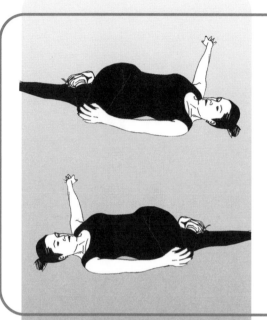

Spinal Twist #2

While lying on your back, bend your right leg, and hook your right toe behind your left knee, as shown. Keep your right arm out straight at a 90-degree angle to maintain your balance. Take your left arm and hand and push down gently on your right knee while keeping your right shoulder blade flat on the ground at all times. Turn your head to look toward your right hand while keeping your head resting on the ground at all times. Keep applying pressure with your left hand and try to get the right knee to touch the ground without the right shoulder blade leaving the ground. Repeat on the other side.

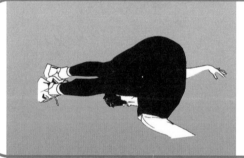

Roll Backs

While lying on your back, roll backward, and balance yourself on your upper shoulders, as shown. Try to extend your legs straight over your forehead and behind you as you hold the stretch.

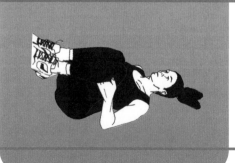

Knees to Chest

While lying on your back, bring both knees up toward your chest, as shown. Grab your right and left legs under your knees with each hand and pull your knees and legs in toward your chest.

Hamstrings—Legs Together

Sit down on the ground with your legs straight, ankles flexed. Bend forward from your hips and reach out toward your toes. Based on your flexibility, grab onto your socks, shoelaces, or toes and hold the stretch. You will feel tension just behind the knees, upper calves, and in the lower back area.

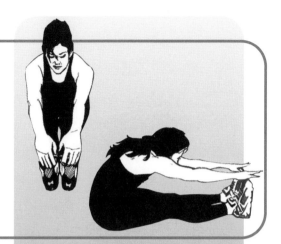

Hamstrings—Legs Apart

Sitting on the ground, with legs straight and apart, bend forward from the hips and reach toward your toes. Based on your flexibility, grab onto your toes or, if this is not possible, your socks or shoelaces.

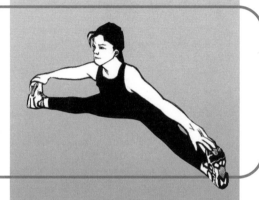

Groin

In a sitting position, pull the soles of your feet together, and grab hold of your ankles. Gently pull your heels toward the groin area. Let your knees relax toward the floor, and gently press your elbows down on your knees to increase the stretch. If you are already flexible in this part of your body, grab your toes and lean forward as far as possible while keeping your back straight.

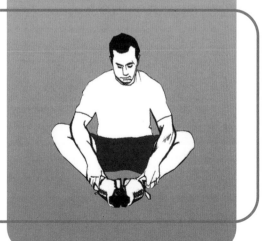

Quadriceps

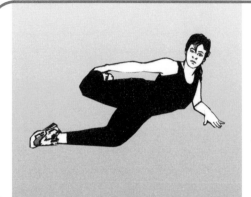

Lie down on your left side and prop yourself up on your left elbow, as shown. Bend your right leg back and grab your right ankle with your right hand. Gently hold your right ankle and bring your leg back toward your buttocks. Hold the position when you feel a comfortable stretch in the front of your thigh. Release slowly, roll over to your right side, and repeat.

Calves #1

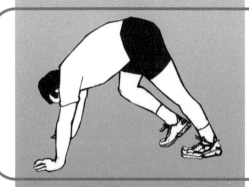

With hands and feet on the ground, make your body into a V shape. With both feet together, bend your right knee and press your left heel toward the ground, stretching your left calf. Repeat on the other side.

Calves #2

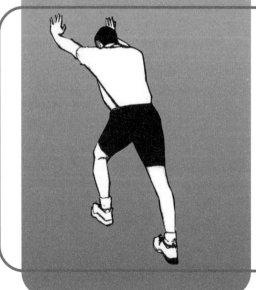

Stand arms-length away from a wall or another solid support. Lean on it with your hands placed shoulder-width apart. Bring your left foot forward, knee bent, while keeping the right leg straight. Lean toward the wall and keep your right heel on the ground while holding the stretch. Switch legs and repeat.

Workload

Lower Body

This exercise strengthens your quadriceps, hamstrings, and buttocks.

Angled Squats

Using the Smith machine, add 30 to 90 lbs. of plates, depending on your current strength level. Do two sets of 10 to 15 reps. Rest 1 to 2 minutes between sets, performing side benders.

Stand erect under the bar with your feet about hip-width apart, your neck comfortably under a neck roll or towel, and your hands gripped wide, as shown. Your feet should be at least 12 inches in front of the rest of your body. Hang onto the bar for stability and balance. With your head up and your back straight throughout the entire movement, squat until your upper thighs are parallel to the floor and then stand up, returning to the starting position. Inhale as you are going down and exhale as you come up. Do not go past a position where your thighs are parallel to the floor when squatting. This exercise can also be done with a narrower stance or a wider stance.

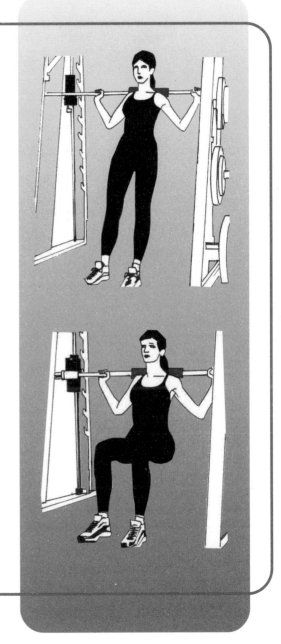

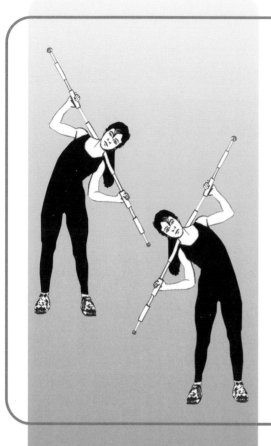

Side Benders

While standing upright, place the aerobic bar on your neck, legs hip-width apart, as shown. Bend to the left side as far as possible without moving your hips or legs. Now bend back to the right side as far as possible. Do not stop in the middle. Keep repeating the movement back and forth at a slow pace until you've caught your breath.

Do not use more than a 4-lb. aerobic bar while performing side benders if you are overweight so as not to build too much muscle under the fat. If you are not overweight, you may use up to a 15-lb. weighted bar to perform side benders.

Upper Body

These exercises strengthen your chest, pectorals, and arms.

Bench Press

Using the incline bench in the flat position or the Olympic bench, do two sets of 40–175 lbs., 10 to 15 reps. Rest 1 to 2 minutes between sets by performing side benders.

Lie on the bench with your feet flat on the floor and hold the barbell about 6 inches wider than shoulder width, as shown. Slowly lower the bar to your chest and then raise the bar up to arms' length. Lower the weight with complete control, making a definite pause at your chest while keeping your head on the bench throughout the entire movement. Do not arch your back at any time and do not raise your hips off the bench. Inhale while lowering the bar and exhale as you raise it. You may also do this exercise with a close grip.

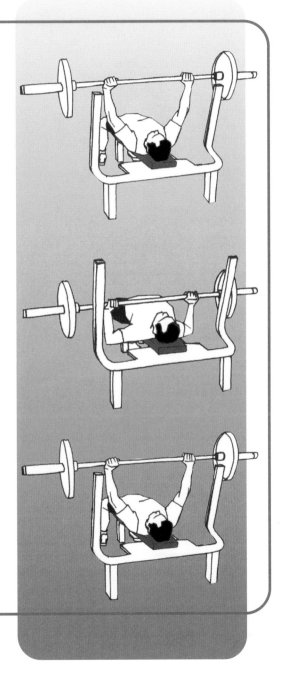

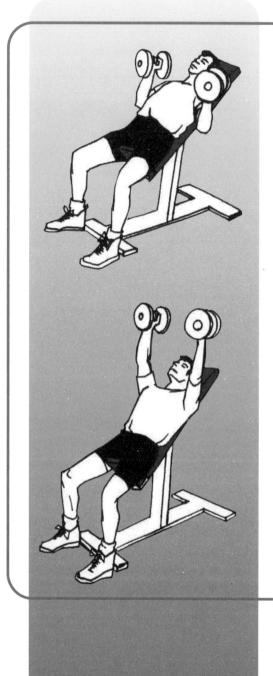

Inclined Dumbbell Press

Using an incline bench with 20–60-lb. dumbbells, depending on your current strength level, do two sets of 10 to 15 reps. Rest 1 to 2 minutes between sets by performing side benders.

Lie on the incline bench with your feet flat on the floor and hold a dumbbell in each hand above your shoulders, palms facing each other, as shown. While inhaling, lower the dumbbells straight down to the sides of your chest, arms close to your sides. Push back up to the starting position while exhaling. Make sure your back is flat and up against the back of the bench at all times; and do not arch your back. This exercise may also be performed with a barbell and weights at each end.

Abdominals/Hips and Legs

These exercises strengthen your core, your upper thighs, and your hips.
To be performed on a firm exercise mat.

Sit-Ups *(Intermediate)*

20 to 40 reps

Lie on your back with your knees bent, feet
flat on the floor with heels up against your
mat, your thumbs clasped with your arms
fully extended, as shown. Slowly raise your
arms (keeping them straight) toward your
knees and perform a full sit-up. Exhale while
sitting up. Slowly lower your body to the
starting position and repeat.

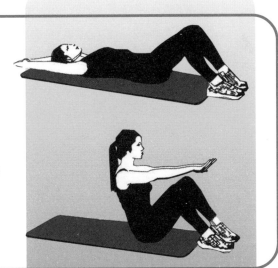

Sit-Ups *(Advanced)*

20 to 40 reps

Lie on your back with your knees bent, feet
flat on the floor with heels up against your
mat, your hands on your ears, as shown.
Slowly raise your body all the way up,
bringing your elbows toward your knees.
Exhale while sitting up. Slowly lower your
body to the starting position and repeat.

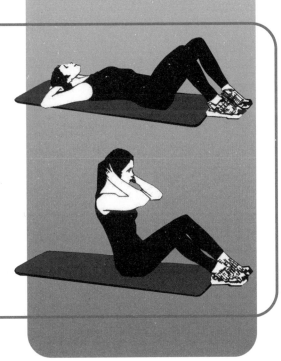

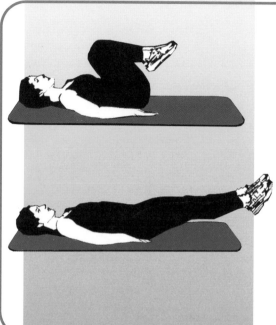

Leg-Outs

**20 reps, rest 30 seconds,
then do another 20 reps**

Lying on your back, with your hands under your buttocks, palms down, bring both knees in toward your chest. Slowly straighten your legs out with toes pointed and repeat. Inhale while bringing your knees toward your chest; exhale as you straighten your legs. Beginners should straighten their legs out at a higher angle. As you get stronger, try to bring your legs lower (about two inches from the ground) while straightening them.

Please note: as your back and abs get stronger, you can move your hands from under your buttocks to behind your neck to intensify the exercise.

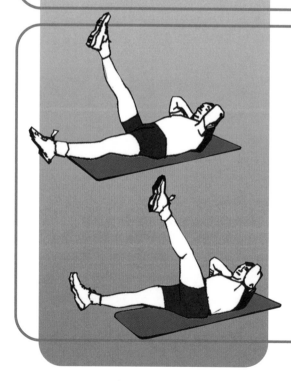

Alternates

**20 reps, rest 30 seconds,
then do another 20 reps**

Lie on your back with your hands under your buttocks, palms down, or clasped behind your neck, as shown, with legs straight, and toes pointed. Raise your right leg to a 90-degree angle; your left leg stays on the floor. Pressing the small of your back into the floor, lower your right leg as you simultaneously lift your left leg to a 90-degree angle. Continuously repeat this scissoring motion.

Please note: as your back and abs get stronger, you can move your hands from under your buttocks to behind your neck to intensify the exercise.

Vertical Scissors

**20 reps, rest 30 seconds,
then do another 20 reps**

(Recommended for women only, unless men's inner and outer thighs are weak or need slimming)

Lie on your back, hands at your sides or next to or under your buttocks, with palms facing down. Raise both legs to a 90-degree angle. Pressing your back into the floor and with toes pointed and legs straight, slowly open your legs as wide as possible and then bring them back together while exhaling, keeping your toes pointed and your legs straight as you repeat the exercise.

Please note: if you possess poor hamstring flexibility, do not attempt this exercise until you have improved that flexibility. As you get stronger, you can intensify this exercise by extending your arms straight out at a 90-degree angle with palms facing down to help maintain your balance.

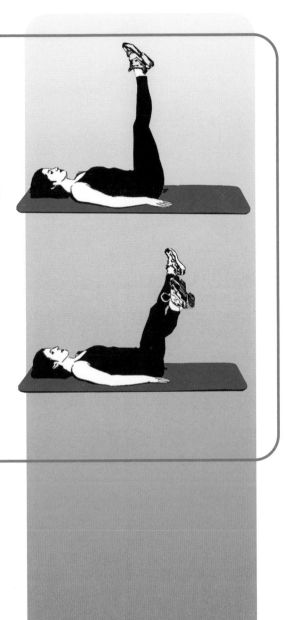

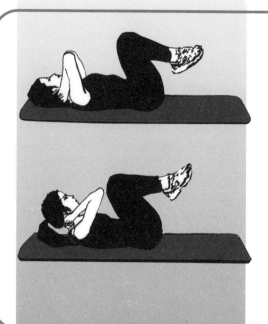

Elbows to Knees

20 reps

Lying on your back, raise your knees and feet toward your chest in a tucked position. Clasp your hands at the base of your neck. Gently curl your upper body, bringing your elbows toward your knees while exhaling. Slowly lower your back and shoulders to the mat while inhaling and repeat. Keep your lower body motionless throughout the entire movement.

Please note: if you cannot touch your elbows to your knees, that's okay. Just reach as far as possible. As you increase your hamstring flexibility, you will eventually be able to touch your elbows to your knees.

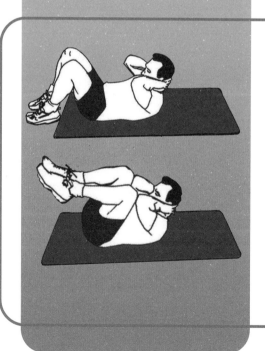

Knees to Elbows

20 reps

Lie on your back with your hands clasped behind the base of your neck. Raise your knees and feet in a tucked position toward your elbows, keeping your lower back pressed against the floor while exhaling. Lower your toes to the ground while inhaling and repeat. Keep the upper half of your body motionless throughout the entire movement.

Please note: if you cannot touch your knees to your elbows, that's okay. Just reach as far as you can. As you increase your hamstring flexibility, you will eventually be able to touch your knees to your elbows.

Leg Lifts

**20 to 30 reps, rest 30 seconds,
then do another 10 to 20 reps**

Lie on your back on the mat with your body fully extended, hands palms down under or next to your buttocks, as shown, with your feet 3 to 8 inches from the ground. Keeping your legs straight and your knees locked, raise your legs as close as possible to a 90-degree angle. Lower your legs, keeping them as straight as possible, to the starting position and repeat. Exhale as you bring your legs up, and inhale as you lower your legs toward the floor. Focus on keeping your back straight throughout the entire movement—do not arch your back. You may also perform leg lifts with your hands behind your neck and/or off a slant board or bench to make it more intense.

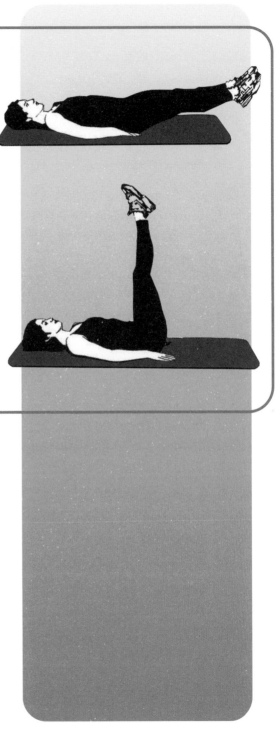

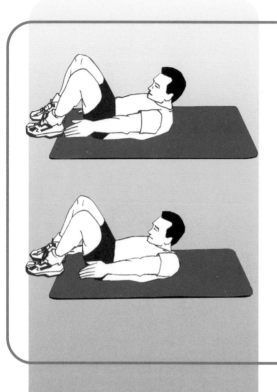

Hand-to-Heel Alternates

30 to 50 reps, rest 30 seconds, and then do another 20 to 40 reps

Lie on your back with your heels flat up against an exercise mat, with your feet 8 to 12 inches apart, as shown. Raise your shoulders slightly off the mat and keep your chin tucked in, as shown. Shift your torso to the left while keeping your lower body as still as possible. Reach with your left fingertips and touch the outside of your left heel. Then, shift back toward your right heel with your right fingertips touching the outside of your right heel, as shown. Do not stop in the middle as you shift back and forth, keeping your shoulder blades off the ground during the entire movement.

Lower Body

This exercise strengthens your quadriceps, hamstrings, and buttocks.

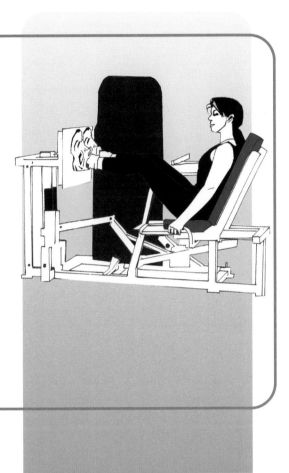

Leg Press

Done on a seated leg-press machine, with 50–200 lbs., depending on your current strength level. Two sets of 10 to 15 reps. Rest 1 to 2 minutes between sets by performing side benders.

Adjust the seat so your upper thighs are nearly vertical to the floor in a contracted position. Hold the handrails under your buttocks and keep your back flat against the back of the bench, as shown. Place your feet on the pad approximately 6 inches apart and, as you exhale, push your legs out until they are almost straight (don't lock your knees). As you inhale, let the weight stack down slowly by bending your knees until it lightly touches the remaining plates and repeat. You may also perform this exercise with your feet wide on the pad.

Upper Body

These exercises strengthen your upper back, chest, forearms, triceps, and wrists. If you don't have access to a chin/dip unit or you cannot perform these exercises, do the exercises described in Option II (page 181).

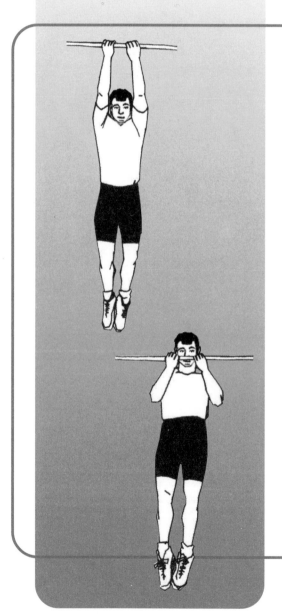

Option I:

Chin-Ups

5 to 12 reps, then 40 to 60 side benders to catch your breath

Use the chinning bar about 6 inches higher off the floor than you can reach (if possible) with your arms extended overhead, your feet dangling in the air, as shown. Hold the bar with your palms facing you about 6 to 8 inches apart. Pull yourself up, trying to get your chin at or above the bar, and then return to the starting position. Try to keep your back slightly hyperextended and do not swing back and forth; exhale while chinning up and inhale while lowering your body down to the starting position. When you lower yourself back down to the starting position, make sure you fully extend your arms so they are as straight as possible. You may also do this exercise with palms facing away from you (pull-ups).

If you need an active rest here, perform 40 to 60 side benders.

Side Benders

While standing upright, place the aerobic bar on your neck, legs hip-width apart, as shown. Bend to the left side as far as possible without moving your hips or legs. Now bend back to the right side as far as possible. Do not stop in the middle. Keep repeating the movement back and forth at a slow pace until you've caught your breath.

Do not use more than a 4-lb. aerobic bar while performing side benders if you are overweight so as not to build too much muscle under the fat. If you are not overweight, you may use up to a 15-lb. weighted bar to perform side benders.

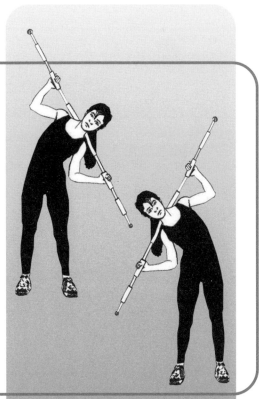

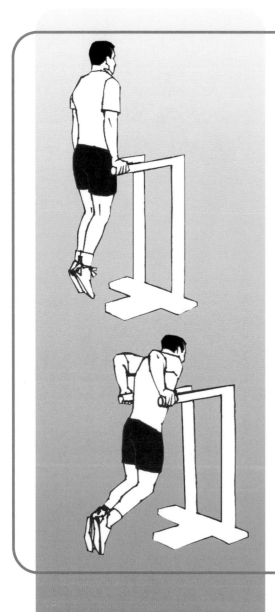

Dips

5 to 12 reps

Hold yourself erect on the bars with your arms straight, as shown. Keep your elbows pressed into your sides; lower your body by bending your elbows. Continue lowering down until your elbows are bent to 90-degree angles, then press back to the starting position. Do not let your body swing back and forth. Exhale as you press up and inhale as you lower your body. You may also perform this exercise while facing outwards, with your back facing the back of the dip unit.

Option II:

Bent-Over Rows

Use either the standard bar or an Olympic bar with 20–60 lbs. of weight added on.

Two sets of 10 to 15 reps

Place the bar in front of you, your knees slightly bent, your hands wider than shoulder-width apart, and bend over with your torso parallel to the floor. Pull the bar straight up toward the lower part of your chest while exhaling. Keeping your lower body still throughout the entire exercise, lower the bar to the starting position while inhaling, and keep your head up and your back as straight as possible. This can also be done with a narrow grip. Maintain moderate speed throughout the entire movement.

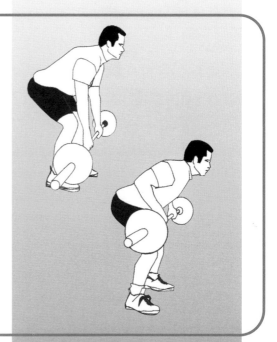

Chair Dips

10 to 20 reps

Position yourself with your arms straight, palms down, holding onto a chair, a bench, or a step. Place your weight on your back heels with your knees slightly bent, as shown, and lower your body, trying to touch the ground lightly with your buttocks. Then push yourself up toward the starting position. Exhale as you push up and inhale as you lower your buttocks toward the ground.

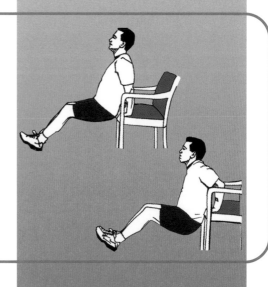

Lower Back

This exercise strengthens your lower back and hamstrings.

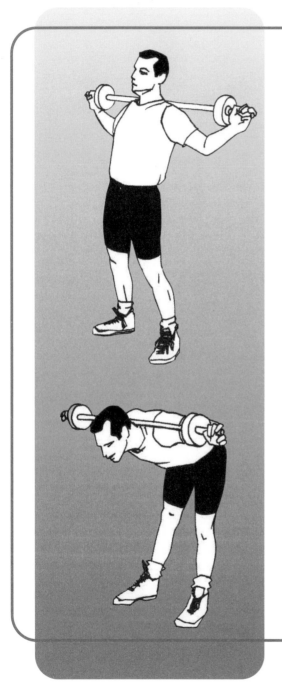

Stiff-Legged Good Mornings

Use a barbell of your choice with 20–60 lbs. of weight added, depending on your current strength level.

Two sets of 15 reps, resting 1 minute between sets

Place the barbell on your shoulders and keep your head up and your back straight. Bend over at the waist, keeping your back flat. Return to the starting position.

Calves

This exercise strengthens your calves, ankles, and feet, and helps improve balance.

Standing Dumbbell One-Legged Toe Raise

Use a dumbbell of your choice, from 20–60 lbs., depending on your current strength level, and a small step.

Two sets of 15 reps, resting one minute between sets

Hold a dumbbell in your right hand, your arm hanging down at your side, palm facing in. Step up on the step with the ball of your right foot, about 2 feet from the wall. Place your left hand against the wall and, keeping your back straight, head up, and right leg locked, place your left foot against your right heel, as shown. Rise up on your right leg, standing as high as possible on the toes of your right foot, and hold the position momentarily, then return to the starting position and repeat. Inhale as you go down and exhale as you push up. Reverse the position and repeat the exercise with your left leg. You may also perform this exercise on a seated calf machine or on a leg press machine.

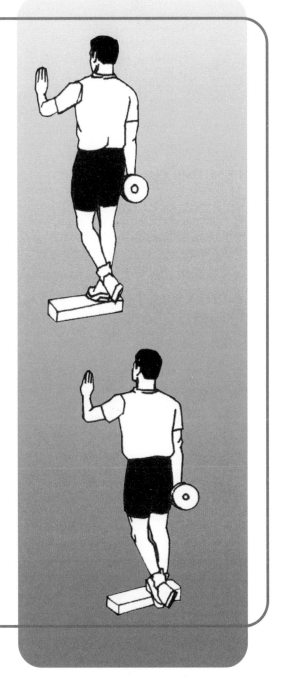

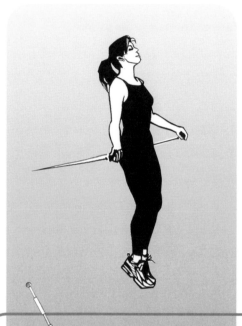

Aerobic Segment

Jump rope for 5 to 10 minutes, fast, then spend 3 minutes biking, walking, jogging, or using any aerobic equipment of your choice—with moderate intensity. If you cannot jump rope, then perform 5 to 10 minutes on your choice of aerobic equipment.

Please note: you may also perform side benders after your aerobic segment or at any time during your workout to catch your breath and/or work on your obliques and range of motion.

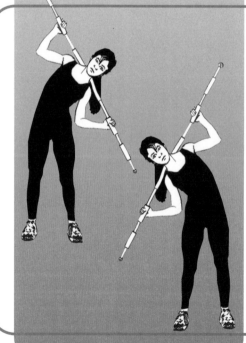

Side Benders

While standing upright, legs hip-width apart, place the aerobic bar on your neck, as shown. Bend to the left side as far as possible without moving your hips or legs. Maintain your stability. Now bend back to the right side as far as possible. Do not stop in the middle. Keep repeating the movement back and forth at a slow pace until you've caught your breath.

Do not use more than a 4-lb. aerobic bar while performing side benders if you are overweight so as not to build too much muscle under the fat. If you are not overweight, you may use up to a 15-lb. weighted bar to perform side benders.

Cool-down

Three minutes of easy biking or walking leisurely.

Program B: Full Body Exercise Regimen

Frequency: 2 days a week.
Duration: 60 to 75 minutes, depending on your current level of fitness.

Warm-up and aerobic segment
Do one of the following for 12 minutes:

- Bike with high tension/resistance at 70+ rpm or 12+ mph.

- Walk at 4+ mph or jog at 6+ mph with extreme hills or incline.

- If you are using an elliptical machine or a cross-trainer, do moderate speed with high resistance and/or incline.

Stretch
Hold each of the following stretches for 30 to 60 seconds. To help you perform your stretches properly and to help you memorize your stretch routine, watch the DVD.

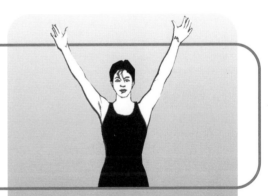

Arm Circles

With arms outstretched, slowly circle your arms backward for five revolutions, and then five revolutions forward. Try to create as big an arc as possible.

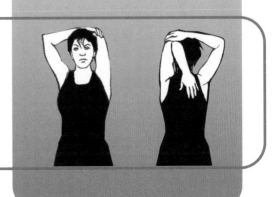

Triceps

With arms overhead, gently pull your left elbow behind your head with your right hand. Hold when you reach a comfortable stretch in the shoulder and upper back. Switch arms and repeat.

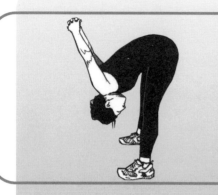

Shoulders and Chest

Grasp your hands behind your back, with palms facing each other. Slightly bend your knees and lift your arms up as you bend forward at the waist. Hold when you feel a comfortable stretch in the shoulders and chest.

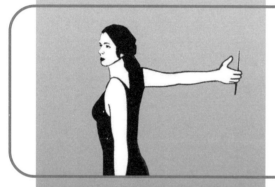

Arms, Upper Back, and Chest

While standing upright, reach behind you with your right arm, keeping it perfectly straight, and grasp onto a door molding or any other immovable object. Now look over your left shoulder and hold the stretch. Switch to your left arm and repeat.

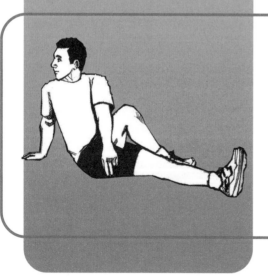

Spinal Twist #1

Sitting on the ground, keep your left leg straight, right arm behind you for support. Cross your right leg over your left knee and place your right foot outside your left knee. With your left hand or elbow on your right knee, slowly twist, and look over your right shoulder while simultaneously pulling your knee in the opposite direction; hold. You will feel pressure in the hip, side, and back. Repeat on the opposite side.

Spinal Twist #2

While lying on your back, bend your right leg, and hook your right toe behind your left knee, as shown. Keep your right arm out straight at a 90-degree angle to maintain your balance. Take your left arm and hand and push down gently on your right knee while keeping your right shoulder blade flat on the ground at all times. Turn your head to look toward your right hand while keeping your head resting on the ground at all times. Keep applying pressure with your left hand and try to get your right knee to touch the ground without the right shoulder blade leaving the ground. Repeat on the other side.

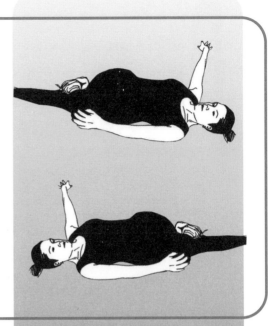

Roll Backs

While lying on your back, roll backward, and balance yourself on your upper shoulders, as shown. Try to extend your legs straight over your forehead and behind you as you hold the stretch.

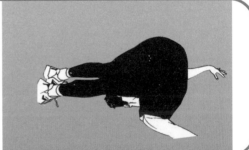

Knees to Chest

While lying on your back, bring both knees up toward your chest, as shown. Grab your right and left legs under your knees with each hand and pull your knees and legs in toward your chest.

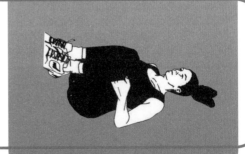

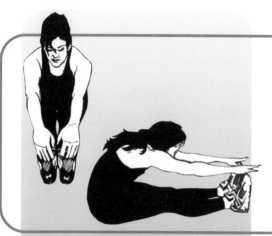

Hamstrings—Legs Together

Sit down on the ground with your legs straight, ankles flexed. Bend forward from your hips and reach out toward your toes. Based on your flexibility, grab onto your socks, shoelaces, or toes and hold the stretch. You will feel tension just behind the knees, upper calves, and in the lower back area.

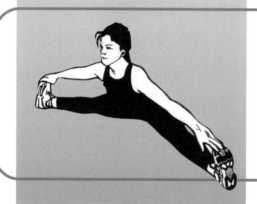

Hamstrings—Legs Apart

Sitting on the ground, with legs straight and apart, bend forward from the hips and reach toward your toes. Based on your flexibility, grab onto your toes or, if this is not possible, your socks or shoelaces.

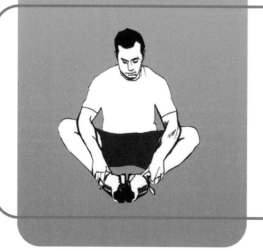

Groin

In a sitting position, pull the soles of your feet together, and grab hold of your ankles. Gently pull your heels toward the groin area. Let your knees relax toward the floor, and gently press your elbows down on your knees to increase the stretch. If you are already flexible in this part of your body, grab your toes and lean forward as far as possible while keeping your back straight.

Quadriceps

Lie down on your left side and prop your-self up on your left elbow, as shown. Bend your right leg back and grab your right ankle with your right hand. Gently hold your right ankle and bring your leg back toward your buttocks. Hold the position when you feel a comfortable stretch in the front of your thigh. Release slowly, roll over to your right side, and repeat.

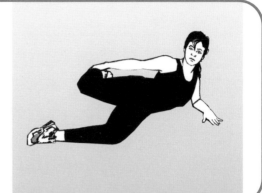

Calves #1

With hands and feet on the ground, make your body into a V shape. With both feet together, bend your right knee and press your left heel toward the ground, stretching your left calf. Repeat on the other side.

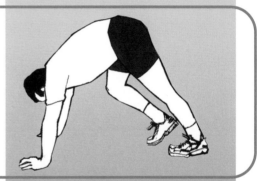

Calves #2

Stand arms-length away from a wall or another solid support. Lean on it with your hands placed shoulder-width apart. Bring your left foot forward, knee bent, while keeping the right leg straight. Lean toward the wall and keep your right heel on the ground while holding the stretch. Switch legs and repeat.

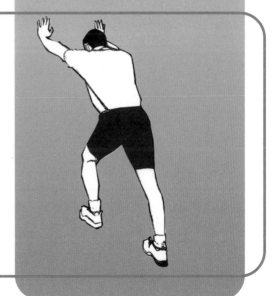

Workload

Lower Body

These exercises strengthen your quadriceps, hamstrings, and buttocks, and help improve your balance.

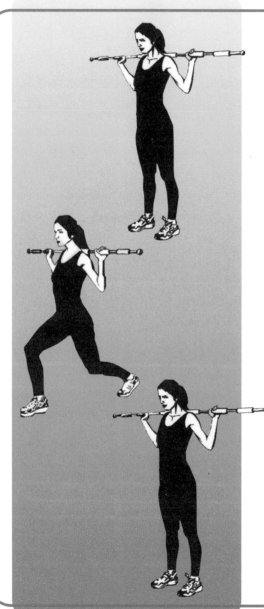

Lunges

Two sets of 15 reps

Place either an aerobic bar, a weighted bar, or a weighted bar with 5–10-lb. plates on each side on the back of your neck across your shoulders, with your hands wider than shoulder-width apart and your feet hip-width apart, as shown. Point your toes straight ahead and step forward with your right leg slightly farther than average stride length, landing right foot heel to toe and coming to a complete stop. Keep your torso erect, inhale, and descend by bending your knees and dropping your hips straight down, stopping short of your left knee touching the ground. While exhaling, push off your right leg and return to the starting position with your feet hip-width apart. Do this exercise one leg at a time and then switch legs and work your left leg.

Step-Ups

Two sets of 15 reps

Stand in front of a bench or step and place either an aerobic bar, a weighted bar, or a weighted bar with 5–10-lb. plates on each side on the back of your neck across your shoulders, with your hands wider than shoulder-width apart and your feet hip-width apart, as shown. While keeping your back straight, place your left leg flat on the bench and step up off the ground with your right while placing all your weight on the left leg and bringing your right leg onto the bench. Lower your right leg to the starting position and repeat. Do this exercise one leg at a time and then switch legs and work your right leg.

As you gain strength and stability, you can step up to a higher bench to increase the intensity.

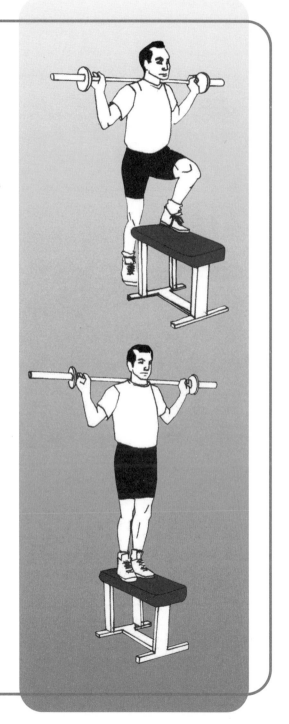

Upper Body
This exercise strengthens your chest, pectorals, upper back, and arms.

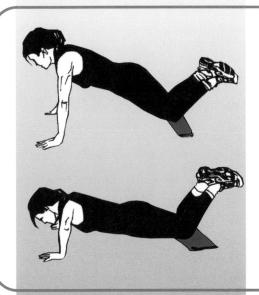

Push-Ups *(Basic)*
Two sets of 15 to 25 reps

On your hands and knees with your ankles crossed, place your knees on a mat or towel with your hands slightly wider than shoulder-width apart, your arms straight, fingers facing forward, and abdominals contracted. While inhaling, lower your chest toward the floor, touching it, and then, while exhaling, push up to the starting position. Keep your back straight and your lower body still throughout the entire exercise.

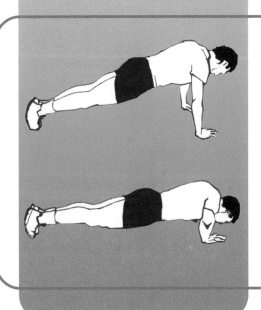

Push-Ups *(Advanced)*
Two sets of 15 to 25 reps

Extend your body on your hands and toes, with your arms straight, and place your hands farther than shoulder-width apart, your fingers facing forward, and abdominals contracted. While inhaling, lower your body toward the floor and lightly touch your chest to the floor. Exhale while pushing up to the starting position and repeat. Do not arch your back or jerk your body during the exercise.

Abdominals/Hips and Legs

These exercises strengthen your core, upper thighs, and hips, and should be performed on a firm exercise mat.

Sit-Ups *(Intermediate)*

20 to 40 reps

Lie on your back with your knees bent, feet flat on the floor with heels up against your mat, your thumbs clasped with your arms fully extended, as shown. Slowly raise your arms (keeping them straight) toward your knees and perform a full sit-up. Exhale while sitting up. Slowly lower your body to the starting position as you inhale, and repeat.

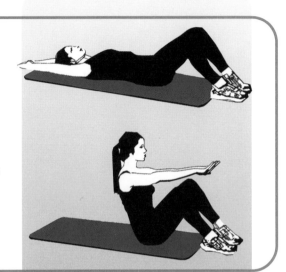

Sit-Ups *(Advanced)*

20 to 40 reps

Lie on your back with your knees bent, feet flat on the floor with heels up against your mat, your hands on your ears, as shown. Slowly raise your body all the way up, bringing your elbows toward your knees. Exhale while sitting up. Slowly lower your body to the starting position as you inhale, and repeat.

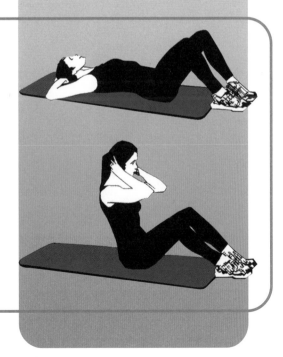

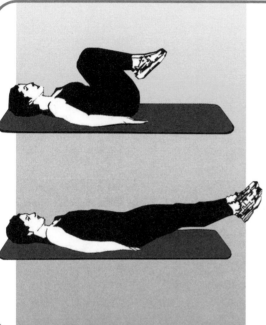

Leg-Outs

**20 reps, rest 30 seconds,
then do another 20 reps**

Lying on your back, with your hands under your buttocks, palms down, bring both knees in toward your chest. Slowly straighten your legs out with toes pointed and repeat. Inhale while bringing your knees toward your chest; exhale as you straighten your legs. Beginners should straighten their legs out at a higher angle. As you get stronger, try to bring your legs lower (about two inches from the ground) while straightening them.

Please note: as your back and abs get stronger, you can move your hands from under your buttocks to behind your neck to intensify the exercise.

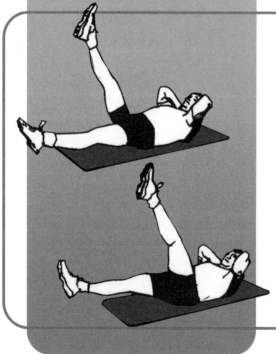

Alternates

**20 reps, rest 30 seconds,
then do another 20 reps**

Lie on your back with your hands under your buttocks, palms down, or clasped behind your neck, as shown, with legs straight, and toes pointed. Raise your right leg to a 90-degree angle; your left leg stays on the floor. Pressing the small of your back into the floor, lower your right leg as you simultaneously lift your left leg to a 90-degree angle. Continuously repeat this scissoring motion.

Please note: as your back and abs get stronger, you can move your hands from under your buttocks to behind your neck to intensify the exercise.

Vertical Scissors

**20 reps, rest 30 seconds,
then do another 20 reps**

(Recommended for women only, unless men's inner and outer thighs are weak or need slimming)

Lie on your back, hands at your sides or next to or under your buttocks, with palms facing down. Raise both legs to a 90-degree angle. Pressing your back into the floor and with toes pointed and legs straight, slowly open your legs as wide as possible and bring them back together while exhaling, keeping your toes pointed and your legs straight as you repeat the exercise.

Please note: if you possess poor hamstring flexibility, do not attempt this exercise until you have improved that flexibility. As you get stronger, you can intensify this exercise by extending your arms straight out at a 90-degree angle with palms facing down to help maintain your balance.

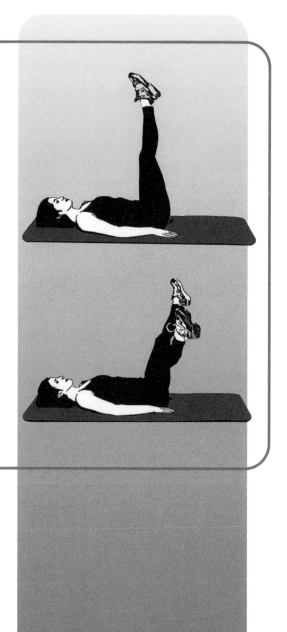

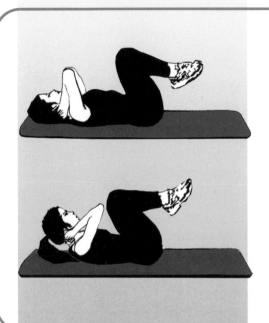

Elbows to Knees

20 reps

Lying on your back, raise your knees and feet toward your chest in a tucked position. Clasp your hands at the base of your neck. Gently curl your upper body, bringing your elbows toward your knees while exhaling. Slowly lower your back and shoulders to the mat while inhaling and repeat. Keep your lower body motionless throughout the entire movement.

Please note: if you cannot touch your elbows to your knees, that's okay. Just reach as far as possible. As you increase your hamstring flexibility, you will eventually be able to touch your elbows to your knees.

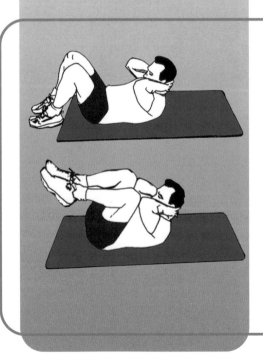

Knees to Elbows

20 reps

Lie on your back with your hands clasped behind the base of your neck. Raise your knees and feet in a tucked position toward your elbows, keeping your lower back pressed against the floor while exhaling. Lower your toes to the ground while inhaling and repeat. Keep the upper half of your body motionless throughout the entire movement.

Please note: if you cannot touch your knees to your elbows, that's okay. Just reach as far as you can. As you increase your hamstring flexibility, you will eventually be able to touch your knees to your elbows.

Leg Lifts

20 to 30 reps, rest 30 seconds, then do another 10 to 20 reps

Lie on your back on the mat with your body fully extended, hands palms down under or next to your buttocks, as shown, with your feet 3 to 8 inches from the ground. Keeping your legs straight and your knees locked, raise your legs as close as possible to a 90-degree angle. Lower your legs, keeping them as straight as possible, to the starting position and repeat. Exhale as you bring your legs up, and inhale as you lower your legs toward the floor. Focus on keeping your back straight throughout the entire movement—do not arch your back. You may also perform leg lifts with your hands behind your neck and/or off a slant board or bench to make the exercise more intense.

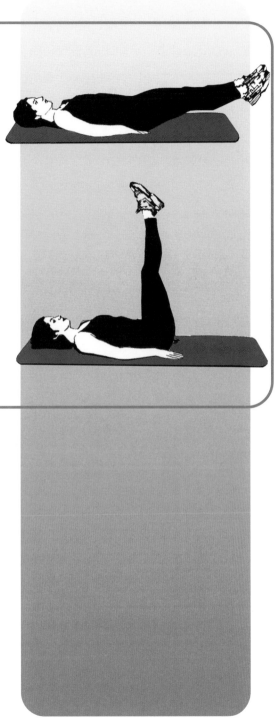

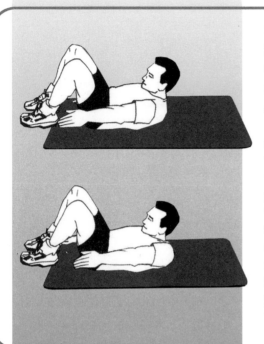

Hand-to-Heel Alternates

30 to 50 reps, rest 30 seconds,
and then do another 20 to 40 reps

Lie on your back with your heels flat up against an exercise mat, your feet 8 to 12 inches apart, as shown. Raise your shoulders slightly off the mat and keep your chin tucked in, as shown. Shift your torso to the left while keeping your lower body as still as possible. Reach with your left fingertips and touch the outside of your left heel. Then, shift back toward your right heel with your right fingertips touching the outside of your right heel, as shown. Do not stop in the middle as you shift back and forth, keeping your shoulder blades off the ground during the entire movement.

Lower Body

These exercises strengthen your quadriceps, hamstrings, and buttocks. For the exercises below, perform one set of leg extensions, then one set of leg curls, rest 1 minute, then repeat leg extensions and leg curls.

Leg Extensions

Two sets of 10 to 15 reps

Depending on your current level of fitness, choose a weight between 40 and 100 lbs. and sit on the machine with your feet under the lower footpads. Hold the seat and raise the weight up until your legs are parallel to the floor. Return to the starting position and repeat in a slow, rhythmic fashion. You may also perform this exercise one leg at a time—with a lighter weight, of course.

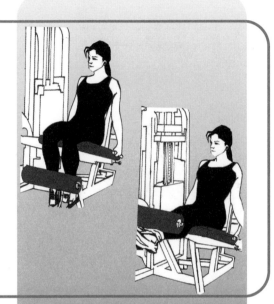

Leg Curls

Two sets of 10 to 15 reps

Choose a weight between 20 and 70 lbs., then lie facedown on the machine and place your heels under the top pad and hold the handles. Curl your legs up until your heels touch your buttocks, or as far as possible without arching your back, and return to the starting position. Repeat in a slow, rhythmic fashion. It is not recommended that you perform this exercise one leg at a time.

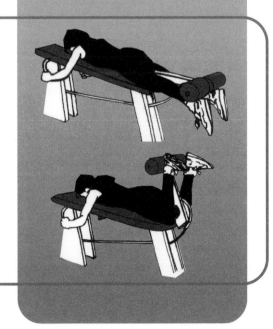

Upper Body

For the exercises below, perform one set of lat pulldowns, then one set of straight arm lat pulldowns, rest 1 to 2 minutes, then repeat lat pulldowns and straight arm lat pulldowns. These exercises strengthen your upper back and shoulders.

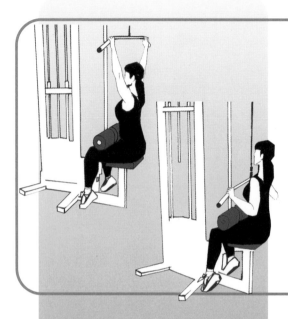

Lat Pulldowns

Two sets of 10 to 15 reps

Choose a weight between 50 and 150 lbs. and sit or kneel and grab the bar with a wide or medium grip with arms extended overhead. Pull the bar straight down until it touches either the back of the neck just above the shoulders or the upper chest. Slowly return to the starting position and repeat. Don't sway your upper body while performing this exercise—concentrate on just moving your arms throughout the entire movement.

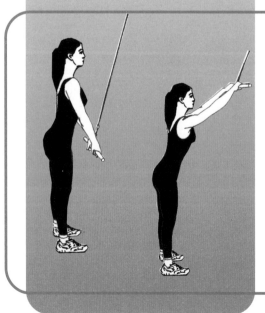

Straight Arm Lat Pulldowns

Two sets of 10 to 15 reps

Choose a weight between 20 and 80 lbs. and stand erect with your knees slightly bent. Grab the bar in front of you with your hands 8 to 16 inches apart. Step back from the machine and pull the bar straight down, in a semicircular motion with your arms straight, until it touches your hips or the top of your thighs. Slowly return the weight to the starting position using the same path. Perform this exercise in a slow, rhythmic fashion and keep upper and lower body still throughout the entire movement.

Lower Body

This exercise strengthens your hamstrings and lower back.

Dead Lifts

Two sets of 15 reps

If you have extremely poor hamstring flexibility or lower back issues, it is recommended that you skip this exercise and work your hamstrings instead by performing two additional sets of leg curls (page 199).

Grip either an aerobic bar, a weighted bar, or a weighted bar with 5–10-lb. plates on each side with your palms facing your body about shoulder-width apart. Hold the bar with your arms fully extended in front of your thighs, your elbows at your sides. Your feet can be either close or wide apart and your knees slightly bent. Keeping the bar close together to the front of your thighs, inhale while you slowly bend at the waist toward your toes and go as far down as possible, trying to touch your toes with the bar, keeping your knees slightly bent. While exhaling, straighten up, keeping your arms fully extended throughout the entire exercise. Squeeze your buttocks as your body straightens up and slightly arch your back at the top of the lift.

Please note: if you possess great hamstring flexibility and have no back issues, you may do this exercise with your legs locked and/or off a step or exercise mat and try to go past your toes, touching the ground with the bar.

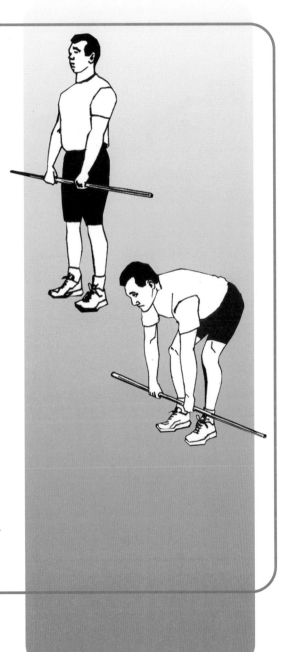

Upper Body
This exercise strengthens your upper back, chest, and arms.

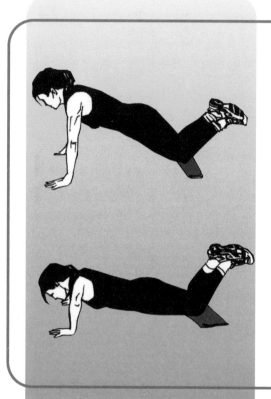

Push-Ups *(Basic)*
Two sets of 15 to 25 reps

On your hands and knees with your ankles crossed, place your knees on a mat or towel with your hands slightly wider than shoulder-width apart, your arms straight, fingers facing forward, and abdominals contracted. While inhaling, lower your chest toward the floor, touching the floor, and then, while exhaling, push up to the starting position. Keep your back straight and your lower body still throughout the entire exercise.

Push-Ups (*Advanced*)

Two sets of 15 to 25 reps

Extend your body on your hands and toes, with your arms straight, and place your hands farther than shoulder-width apart, your fingers facing forward, and abdominals contracted. While inhaling, lower your body toward the floor and lightly touch your chest to the floor. Exhale while pushing up to the starting position and repeat. Do not arch your back or jerk your body during the exercise.

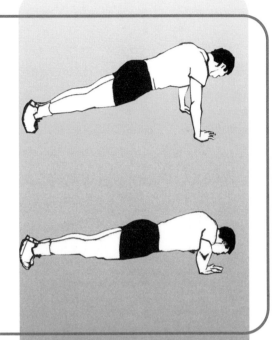

Aerobic Segment

Jump rope for 5 to 10 minutes, fast, then spend 3 minutes biking, walking, jogging, or using any aerobic equipment of your choice—with moderate intensity. If you cannot jump rope, then perform 12 minutes on your choice of aerobic equipment.

Please note: you may also perform side benders after your aerobic segment or at any time during your workout to catch your breath and/or work on your obliques and range of motion.

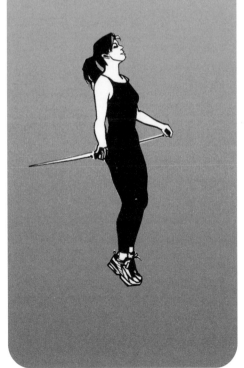

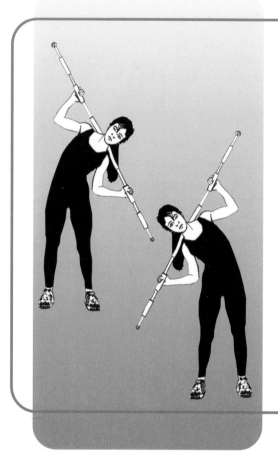

Side Benders

While standing upright, legs hip-width apart, place the aerobic bar on your neck, as shown. Bend to the left side as far as possible without moving your hips or legs. Maintain your stability. Now bend back to the right side as far as possible. Do not stop in the middle. Keep repeating the movement back and forth at a slow pace until you've caught your breath.

To keep from building up too much muscle under the fat, do not use more than a 4-lb. aerobic bar while performing side benders. As you get stronger, increase the weight of the bar as you perform side benders.

Cool-down
Three minutes of easy biking or walking leisurely.

As you strengthen your body, you will become more efficient with your workouts and your club speed will increase, resulting in more distance. You will be less fatigued in general for day-to-day activities, and a round of golf will not only become more enjoyable, but easier as well.

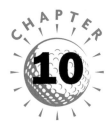

CHAPTER 10

Additional Exercises and Helpful Golf Tips

Your workouts will allow you to improve your overall fitness level, but you may need to supplement these workouts with additional exercises specifically targeting areas that are used during your golf game. For instance, your forearms and wrists may be weak and you may need to strengthen them so that you can grip the club properly on your backswing or power the ball out of the deep rough. Or, perhaps you need to work on your obliques (those muscles located on the sides of your stomach), which are critical for helping you turn and swing through the ball with more power. Here are some additional exercises you can add to your current fitness routine. You may do any or all of these exercises during your routine or separately at another time. Make sure you rest at least one day before repeating any of the exercises outlined here.

Upper Body

Wrists, Forearms, and Hands

You can perform these exercises either on the days you don't do your upper body routine or after you've completed your upper body exercises. Don't do any of these exercises on the days when you play a round of golf until after you've completed your round.

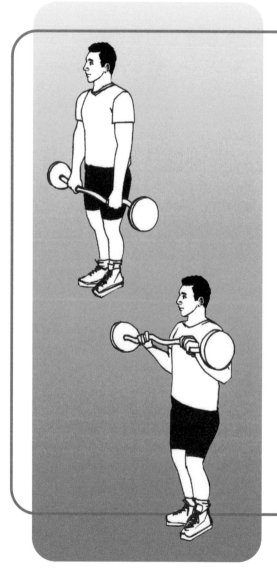

Reverse Curls

Three sets of 10 to 20 reps, with 2 minutes of rest between sets

Holding the Olympic bar with 5–10 lbs. of weight added on, stand with your feet about hip-width apart. Let both arms hang down in front of your body, fully extended, with your palms facing in toward your body. Next, lift the bar upward. Slowly return to the starting position and repeat. Be sure to keep your elbows at your sides throughout the exercise.

Wrist Roll-Ups

Three sets of 15 to 20 reps, with 2 minutes of rest between sets

Hold the weighted bar out in front of you with palms facing down. Twist your hands up so palms are facing forward.

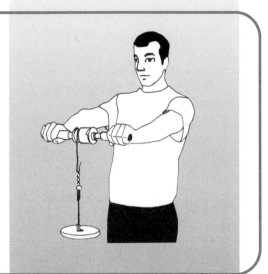

Hand Grips

Using a tennis ball or spongy-type ball or one of these grip strengtheners, squeeze the hand grips as tightly as you can, release, and repeat for as many reps as you can.

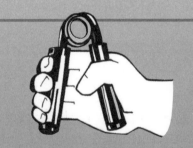

More Wrist Exercises

A soft-gel ball is great to have with you at all times—squeezing it repeatedly strengthens your hands and wrists, and it also burns calories throughout the day. Also, chin-ups are very good for building hand and wrist strength.

Core and Back

These exercises strengthen your obliques and your lower back.

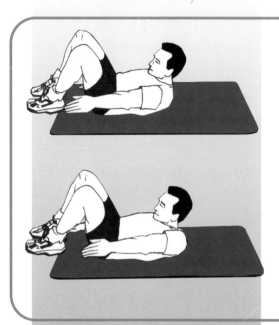

Hand-to-Heel Alternates

Three sets of 20 to 50 reps, with 1 minute between sets

This exercise works the obliques, which help you complete your swing.

Lie on your back on an exercise mat and place your feet approximately 12 to 18 inches from your buttocks, as shown. Lift your shoulders and keep your chin tucked in, as shown. Shift your torso to the right and touch the outside of your right heel. Then shift to your left side and touch your left heel. Alternate back and forth on each side. To make this exercise more intense, bring your heels farther away from your buttocks.

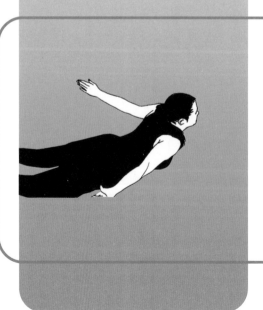

Chest Tilts

This exercise works the midsection and the lower portion of your back.

Lie on your stomach on an exercise mat or soft surface, bring your arms out to the side, and arch your back while lifting your chest off the surface as high as you can (your pelvic area remains on the ground). Try to hold the "up" position, as illustrated, for 30 to 60 seconds, then return your upper body to the surface. Repeat 5 to 10 times, resting 1 minute between sets.

Lower Body

Leg Tilts

This exercise works your hamstrings and gluteus (buttocks), which help with stability and balance.

Lie on your stomach on an exercise mat or soft surface and place your arms in front of you on the surface, as illustrated. Tilt your right leg up as high as possible while keeping your pelvis on the ground and hold for 30 to 60 seconds. Lower your leg and repeat on the left side. Repeat 5 to 10 times, resting 30 seconds between sets.

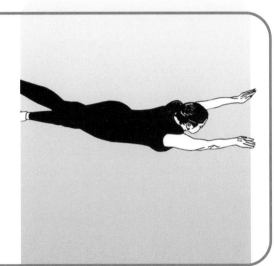

Side Benders

Side benders are great to intersperse throughout your workouts whenever you need to rest between exercises. They really work your lower abdominal muscles, which ease the stress when you turn for your wood or iron shots. One other thing you can do to increase your swing speed is to practice swinging a weighted golf club.

While standing upright, legs hip-width apart, place the aerobic bar on your neck, as shown. Bend to the left side as far as possible without moving your hips or legs. Maintain your stability. Now bend back to the right side as far as possible. Do not stop in the middle. Keep repeating the movement back and forth at a slow pace until you've caught your breath.

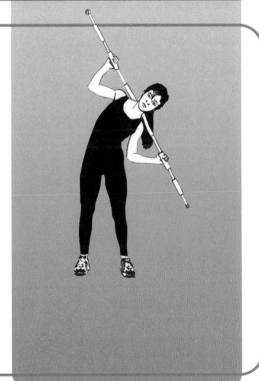

Fitness Tips for the Days You Play Golf

- **Spend 20–30 minutes warming up, stretching, and hitting some balls.**

- Warming up protects your body from injury and keeps a medical condition from worsening. It also helps you adjust faster to inclement weather.

- If you have to wait longer than usual between holes, especially on chilly days, keep your body moving, stretch, or chip balls (if that's allowed). That will keep you loose and relaxed.

When and When Not to Exercise

When should you exercise during the golf season? If you live where the seasons change and there are colder months when you cannot play golf, it is obviously easier to schedule your workout days because you're not tempted to get out on the course. On the other hand, if you live in a climate where you're able to play golf year-round, it's a little bit tougher to pick and choose when to do your formal workouts, when to practice at the range, and when to fit in your rounds of golf. Those who can only play golf seasonally exercise a lot more during the colder months but virtually abandon their workouts and exercise a lot less during the golf season. That type of schedule poses three problems. First, you become an in-shape and then an out-of-shape person, and you can't really achieve either your fitness or your weight loss goals because you are seesawing up and down. Second, toward the end of the summer season, your fitness level is so low that you cannot take advantage of all that hard work you put in during the winter months because you have nothing left in reserve. Third, you cannot significantly improve your distance and scoring during the golf season. Do you think any of the top professional golfers on any of the tours only work out during their "off season"?

Year-round golfers tend to exercise less frequently during the week but don't let as much time elapse between workouts; they also do not work out as long (duration) each time they do work out. Whether you play golf year-round or seasonally, try to find a fitness program you can stick with and perform regularly year-round. The more fit you are, the better you will golf and the more you will enjoy your game.

Putting It All Together

So when should you exercise, how frequently, how intensely, and what type of exercise routine should you do? Below are some guidelines for both year-round golfers and seasonal golfers to keep in mind when deciding when to golf and when to exercise.

Do not perform a full body fitness routine before playing eighteen holes unless you have been exercising for years and you are very fit. Until you fine-tune your fitness routine and are in good shape, whenever possible, wait until after your golf round to perform a full body or vigorous fitness routine.

You may, however, perform a full body routine after your round, provided that you avoid alcohol until after you've exercised and played golf.

If you want to work out on days you play eighteen holes of golf, you may perform an aerobic, stretch, and abdominals routine, as long as you are somewhat in shape and riding in a golf cart. If you are overweight or out of shape and will be walking eighteen holes that day, use common sense as to whether to exercise that day, depending on how you feel.

You should warm up for a few minutes and then stretch every day you hit golf balls at the range or play a round of golf.

On the days you go to the range, if you perform a full-body exercise routine beforehand, hit your short irons (unless you are used to exercising often and are in good shape).

Below is a sample of a typical one-week calendar of fitness, golf-range hitting, and playing golf that can help you reach your golf goals—to play as well and as often as you like.

Depending on your goals, each week you should perform three full body fitness routines and one to two aerobic/abs routines and set up one to two golf range dates. If you are overweight, you need five days of exercise. If you are not overweight but want to strengthen your body, you only need to perform three full body routines per week.

If you can only play golf seasonally, you might want to consider purchasing a small golf mat and golf net to hit golf balls during your off season.

Remember, this is only a guide. The better conditioned and the more fit you become, the easier it will be to work out before or

Golfer's Sample Calendar

Monday
Full body fitness routine

Tuesday
Rest day

Wednesday
Full body fitness routine

Thursday
Golf range and aerobic/abs routine

Friday
Full body fitness routine

Saturday
Golf round

Sunday
Golf range and aerobic/abs routine

after a round of golf or to hit golf balls at the range at any time. Just as you need to practice and play golf often in order to get your muscles used to the golf swings, you also need to get your body used to working out. This is how you form what is known as *muscle memory*. Muscle memory is the common term for neuromuscular facilitation, the process of the neuromuscular system memorizing motor skills. By repeating the movements of your golf swing, you will increase your level of accuracy.

Mental Fitness

That brings me to perhaps the most important aspect of being fit—mental fitness, and how it carries over to your golf game. When you're fit, you can play a round of golf any time. At the end of a round, you hardly feel any physical effects. You're able to get your swing into a groove more easily and you're able to hit the golf ball farther and farther as the round progresses. Being fit also helps you with your putting because you can stay focused for longer periods of time, stay calmer and more steady, and control your body (and nerves), which enables you to swing with pinpoint accuracy. Being physically fit and possessing good balance can help you on awkward or severe uphill or downhill lies. You shouldn't feel tired after eighteen holes of golf, whether you've walked the course or not—unless, of course, you're unfit! As you become fit, you'll enjoy each round of golf more and more.

CHAPTER 11

Fueling Yourself for Fitness and Golf

How often do you complete nine holes of golf and head straight to the halfway house, your mouth watering for that legendary hot dog? Hey, don't get me wrong, every once in a while there's nothing wrong with a hot dog, a hamburger, even an occasional dessert.

I don't need to harp on how much heavier both adults and children are today, worldwide. Having consulted with thousands of golfers and nongolfers about weight loss over the years, I have observed that, overall, golfers tend to be a bit heavier. The reason for this might be that golfers typically substitute golfing/walking for a formal exercise routine, and they don't normally work out on the days they play golf. Eating properly is essential not only for general good health and maintaining a healthy weight, but it's also critical for sustaining energy for your workouts and for playing golf.

Healthy Eating Tips for Golfers

Here are some guidelines to help you develop good eating habits:

- Don't skip meals; you'll overeat at your next meal and this will lead to weight gain.
- Eat smaller meals and less food on the days you don't exercise.
- Eat smaller meals on the days you only play golf, if you ride in a golf cart.
- Prepare snacks and lunch (if applicable) on the days you are playing golf, especially if the course where you're playing does not offer healthy food choices.
- If you are on a specific diet for either medical reasons or weight loss, make sure you prepare foods ahead of time to take with you while playing golf.
- Bring extra water with you when golfing on hot days.
- Avoid alcohol while playing golf.
- Avoid drinking excessive amounts of soda or coffee while playing golf—they will dehydrate you.
- If you're playing golf early in the morning, eat a small meal before you go.
- Bananas are great snacks and will give you energy if you're in between meals and feel hungry.

- Yogurt is also a great snack food that can be made into a meal when mixed with fruit or granola.
- Eat carbohydrates before you exercise and/or play golf.
- Keep in mind that weight loss/gain is simply an equation of calories in versus calories out: fewer calories in than out equals weight loss; more calories in than out equals weight gain.
- Consult with your healthcare professional or doctor before you decide to take supplements of any kind.
- Avoid diets that are too severe and those that do not consist of a well-balanced mix of fats, proteins, and carbohydrates.

Here are some healthy meal suggestions for a day of golf.

Breakfast (1–2 hours pregame):

- Egg-white omelet with nonfat cheese, 2 slices whole-wheat toast/jam, piece of fruit
- Toasted whole-wheat bread or an English muffin topped with 1 oz. nonfat cheese, piece of fruit
- Milkshake made with skim milk, nonfat fruit yogurt, and fresh fruit
- High fiber cereal with skim milk and fresh fruit (bran cereals available in miniboxes)
- A piece of fresh fruit with a cup of non-fat yogurt and 2–3 graham crackers
- Yogurt with bran cereal and raisins
- Instant oatmeal with $1/2$ banana and minibox of raisins (can add cottage cheese)
- Power bar

Drink Gatorade five minutes prior to starting the round and throughout the day if you don't have time to eat before starting.

Snacks:

Try to snack often and bring easy-to-carry snacks. If possible, keep a cooler in your cart.
- Mixed fruit
- 1 minibox raisins or 7 dried apricot halves
- 1 cup popcorn
- 2 teaspoons sesame seeds or another favorite nut
- Store-bought trail mix, mostly dried fruit (small portion)
- Cereal bar or power bar
- Fruit: banana, oranges, berries
- Individual box of high-fiber cereal with minibox of raisins
- Sports drink, such as Gatorade, mixed with water

Salads:

Salads are usually available back at the restaurant or clubhouse after your golf game. Make a salad the base, and top it with lean fish or chicken. Eat a salad by itself as a meal or as an appetizer. The choices for salads are almost endless, and what I like best is that they fill us up without filling us out. Here are a few of my favorite reasons to enjoy salads as a way of eating:

- They can be made with raw or cooked foods, hot or cold, and you can throw in those leftovers.
- They can be made with a foundation of salad greens and vegetables, which are filling (high volume), take a long time to eat, and can be much lower in calories than traditional meals (though do be mindful of the calories in salad dressing).
- Salads are packed with vitamins, minerals, and disease-fighting phytochemicals. They also have lots of fiber.

- Salads can feed our senses with a variety of colors and textures.

- Salad-making can be fun, creative, tasty, and help maintain weight.

Salads are a great way to eat more like a vegetarian without becoming one. You can use different types of greens, vegetables, and even fruits. You can add in grilled foods, such as grilled chicken, grilled veggies, and grilled seafood. You can eat a salad as an appetizer or as a main course. So, if you're looking for easy, nutrient-dense, healthy, filling, low-calorie meals, start with salads.

To help educate and motivate you to eat healthier so you have more energy to become more fit, lose weight, or play better golf, I've enlisted the expertise of one of America's leading nutritionists and a weight management specialist, June Lay, president of Junefit.com. Together, we've assembled the most important specifics on nearly every major aspect of nutrition. Below, you'll find suggestions to improve the way you look, feel, and function on a daily basis. If you'd like to contact June, email her at june@junefit.com.

General Healthy Eating Tips

Are we healthy yet? Or, to be more precise, are we eating healthy yet? And what does healthy eating mean? Well, I think it depends on who you talk to, or what expert you're listening to. I recommend that you eat often; start early, with breakfast; and combine small amounts of protein with your carbohydrate foods. I call these the "tools" of eating for health, energy, and weight loss. But let's take a closer look at what would be considered healthy eating habits by most experts (it's not only about your weight!). If you spend a little more time on what you should add to your diet, rather than what you should cut out, I believe you might find yourself eating healthy more often.

So, do you:

- Eat at least three different fruits a day

- Eat at least three to five different vegetables per day (in a variety of colors, including dark green leafy ones and also cruciferous veggies)

- Eat a meal that is totally vegetarian once a week

- Eat fish instead of red meat or poultry at least twice a week

- Eat or drink a low-fat dairy product such as yogurt or milk two to three times a day (or a nondairy, calcium-fortified product)

- Eat whole grains instead of white flour foods (this includes high-fiber cereals, brown rice, etc.) almost every day

- Eat a nutrient-dense snack instead of a high-calorie, nonnutrient snack (popcorn instead of M&Ms, for instance) more than 50 percent of the time

- Substitute a low-fat alternative for foods high in fat (jelly instead of butter, or chicken stock instead of oil in cooking) more than 50 percent of the time?

- Are you using healthy, monounsaturated fats, such as olive oil instead of butter, when you do use fat to cook

If you remember to apply these healthy eating principles most of the time, then you can enjoy other choices some of the time without feeling guilty. Feeling overwhelmed by the list? Start small and see how the healthy habit grows!

Live Longer by Eating Healthy

Live longer by eating healthy. Sound simple? Studies continually report a high positive correlation between eating healthy and living longer, so the way you eat impacts your longevity and well-being.

Our lifestyle habits are the most important components of longevity that we have control over. How we feed our bodies can make a difference in our health (short and long term), energy levels, mood, and mental performance. What we eat regularly is a lifestyle factor.

While there is no single way of eating that is perfect, and there is no single way of eating that works for all of us, there are a few guidelines that will help us all.

Here are a few "eat healthy" lifestyle questions to ask yourself:

- Did I start my day with some fuel (that is, breakfast)?
- Have I eaten something every few hours, even just a quick, healthy snack?
- Have I balanced my intake of healthy, high-nutrient food with just a few low-nutrient-type foods?
- Have I had enough water to hydrate myself and compensate for any coffee, soda, or alcoholic drinks I've had?

- Have I cut back on fats and sugars and added a few more fruits and veggies?
- Did I only eat a sweet treat after "real food"?
- Can I cut my portions by just 10 percent most of the time (studies show that this the only variable, in and of itself, that may increase life span!)?

Feed the Brain

Is there a brain-food connection, and if so, what food will enhance the brain's performance? The brain controls and regulates all our voluntary and involuntary physical functions, as well as the mysterious functioning of our minds. Proper brain nutrition, according to experts, corresponds directly to the intake of carbohydrates, fats, and proteins, so we should reconsider diets that eliminate or drastically reduce any one type of food (I couldn't resist, since so many of us are carb-starved these days!). All those nutrients provide the brain with the raw materials to protect it, power it, and keep it functioning at its best.

The most important brain foods are:

- **Carbohydrates.** Complex carbohydrates, such as those found in starches, grains, vegetables, and fruits (fruits are technically simple carbs), give the brain the raw material for glucose. Glucose is the main fuel that powers the brain—brain cells use glucose for energy. The brain cannot store glucose the way muscles can, so we need a steady supply of this fuel. This means that if you haven't eaten all day, or you're on a restricted carbohydrate diet, you may find yourself craving sweets, feeling fatigued or moody, or just not functioning at your best (you may not even be aware of your lowered abilities). Carbohydrates are also the primary source of most vitamins, minerals, and phytochemicals (including antioxidants), which protect the brain from premature aging and disease.

- **Fats.** Yes, fats! Fats, the essential fatty acids found mainly in our polyunsaturated and monounsaturated fats (fats found in coldwater fish, shellfish, vegetables, nuts, and seeds), provide the brain with the raw materials to maintain brain-cell membrane integrity and functioning. The journal of *Neurobiology of Learning and Memory* reported a study done on rats (their brains function much like ours), in which they were fed a diet consisting of 40 percent fat (similar to what most Americans eat) and lost cognitive functioning. The study found that when the diet was high in saturated fat as opposed to unsaturated fat, the rats suffered more impairment—their learning and memory functioning were significantly reduced. Saturated fat can clog arteries by causing a buildup of plaque that eventually reduces blood flow. And we don't need to guess what reduced blood flow means to our thinking ability! So, let's eat our fats, but let's be choosy about where they come from.

- **Proteins.** Proteins provide the raw materials for those vital brain chemicals known as neurotransmitters. For instance, when you eat a piece of lean meat that contains tryptophan, you enable your body to make the well-known neurotransmitter serotonin by providing it with needed amino acids. Lean meats, such as chicken, fish, and turkey, provide the same amino acids as higher-fat meats without the dangerous saturated fats.

- **Water and Exercise.** Water is the primary component of blood, which carries all vital nutrients to the brain. Exercise increases circulation and therefore increases the blood supply to the brain.

So, at your next meal, remember that you're feeding your brain, as well as your body. Although the brain averages about 2 percent of your body weight, it uses more than 20 percent of your energy, and about half of the blood sugar floating in your blood vessels. In sports, feeding the brain becomes just as important as feeding the body. Golf requires tremendous mental concentration and focus.

Eat Some Protein with Your Carbs

It is important to combine different types of foods at each meal or snack. Combining protein foods with carbohydrate foods can actually help you to lose weight, while also maintaining blood sugar levels in an optimal range. This is how people with diabetes are instructed to eat. While most of us do not need to worry about our blood sugar level falling too low or rising too high, we are still physically and mentally affected when our blood sugar level falls to the low end of normal. Ever experience any of these symptoms after not eating for a long period of time or a short time after eating a high-sugar food?

- Fatigue
- Moodiness/irritability
- Cravings for sweets

- Hunger leading to overeating

- An uncontrollable urge to eat

Why? Your brain requires a steady supply of fuel; without it, even the healthiest among us will experience these symptoms. The brain only uses glucose—this is a sugar in its simplest form, so sugar is not an enemy. But if you eat a high-sugar snack, a quick fix can become a crash. This can lead to sugar cravings and binges at the end of the day. How to minimize this? Eat like a diabetic.

Eating like a diabetic means eating a food high in protein along with a food high in carbohydrates, such as a slice of low-fat cheese with half a bagel. What will this do? The protein in the cheese will slow down the digestive process, which will raise blood sugar more slowly, supplying a steady flow of energy. Add this to our "eating often" program and we'll feel better, have more energy, eat less junk food, and most of us will need less food overall, especially at the end of the day. This supplies a steady flow of sugar (glucose) to the blood to feed our cells and our brain. Combining foods is a good thing, so don't fall prey to gimmicks (like diets that eliminate carbs, for instance). And when a little fat is added to a meal, it will help slow down the digestive/absorption process as well.

Healthy Eating Includes Grains

Are we eating our grains? According to studies reported by the American Dietetic Association, we are not! According to a recent report in the *Journal of the ADA*, Americans are consuming far fewer than the recommended three servings of a grain food per day. In fact, most of us are consuming less than one serving a day.

Looking at the USDA Food Guide Pyramid, we are supposed to consume between six and eight grain/starch food servings a day, and three of these should come from whole grains.

Based on scientific evidence, regular consumption of whole-grain foods reduces rates of coronary heart disease and several forms of cancer.

Here's why:

- Whole grains contain hundreds of phytochemicals, those nonnutrient compounds that help fight disease.

- Whole grains also contain many important vitamins and minerals, such as several B vitamins, vitamin E, and selenium.

- Whole grains contain fiber.

Foods that contain whole grains include:

- Cereals such as Wheaties, Cheerios, whole grain Total, Raisin Bran, Grape Nuts, Shredded Wheat, and oatmeal.

- Whole-wheat bread, whole-wheat pita, whole-wheat crackers, popcorn (air-popped), wild rice, brown rice, bulgur, whole-wheat pastas, and wheat berries.

Start the day with a healthy cereal, or add some cereal to your yogurt. Have a healthy turkey sandwich on whole-wheat bread for lunch, and a few whole-wheat crackers with an ounce of low-fat cheese for an afternoon snack. Prefer some pasta or rice? Try wild rice or whole-wheat pasta.

Fiber, the Nonnutrient Nutrient

Fiber is a general term for the structural parts of plants that are not digestible and absorbable to humans (although some fibers are partially digested in the colon by bacteria). For this reason, fiber is not considered a nutrient. However, fiber has been proven to be as valuable for our health as nutrients. There are two types of fiber—soluble and insoluble—and while many plant foods contain both, one type is usually predominant in each food. Soluble fiber forms a gel when mixed with liquid, while insoluble fiber does not. Insoluble fiber passes through the intestines largely intact.

Wheat, whole grains, and most vegetables contain insoluble fiber; these act as natural laxatives. They are not completely digested and absorbed, and so add weight and bulk to the waste material in our large intestine. This increases the transit time of solid foods through the intestines (a healthy thing), which means they usually help us to eliminate more often. (We also need to drink more water when we eat more fiber; otherwise we may experience constipation.) Other benefits of insoluble fiber include:

- Slowing down the digestion of other starches, thereby delaying rapid glucose absorption into the blood.

- Helping to prevent digestive ailments, such as diverticulosis, irritable bowel syndrome, and constipation by adding weight and increasing transit time, thus lowering internal pressure through the large intestine.

- Helping to lower colon cancer risk by increasing the removal of solid waste material from the body, thus protecting from bacterial buildup.

Soluble fiber, the type of fiber found in oatmeal, barley, apples, citrus fruits, and legumes, slows down the transit time of food as well. Soluble fiber also helps to decrease your blood sugar level after eating (a good thing, especially for diabetics), and lowers blood cholesterol levels. If you're looking for long-lasting energy, lowered

cholesterol levels, and that feeling of food sticking to your ribs, then a small bowl of oatmeal with fruit is the way to go.

A high-fiber diet can help you maintain and even lose weight. Studies report that people who eat high-fiber foods consume an average of 150 fewer calories daily than those who do not. This may not sound like that many calories, but over the course of a year it can add up to ten pounds. Fiber can also help prevent gallstones and metabolic disorders, including type II diabetes. And don't forget all the good vitamins, minerals, and disease-fighting phytochemicals in these foods. For a nonnutrient nutrient, fiber sure has a lot of healthy properties!

Become a Vegetarian

Become a vegetarian for one day a week, so you're forced to eat more fruits and veggies. Choose whole-grain products, vegetables, and fruits as your main source of food on that day. Each vegetable and fruit has its own profile of "phytochemicals" and the American Institute for Cancer Research says, "The discovery of phytochemical-protective substances in food is new. Each phytochemical seems to have a unique role in cancer protection."

These foods provide most of the vitamins, minerals, phytochemicals, and complex carbohydrates that we need for energy and to fight disease. They are naturally low in fat, high in fiber, and they're filling. Now, an important factor in keeping these foods "high in nutrient density" is to prepare them by using a low-fat method; otherwise they will become "high in caloric density" instead.

You're more likely to add more plant foods to your diet on nonvegetarian days if you practice being a vegetarian even for only one day a week. (I've found that the more veggies I eat, the more I want to eat!) By doing this, you'll automatically increase your fiber intake. Fiber is only found in plant foods like whole-grain breads, beans, vegetables, and fruits. Plant foods also lower the risk for heart disease, endocrine disorders (such as diabetes), and some cancers. Other essential nutrients, such as B vitamins in grains and legumes, have been shown to play a role in the prevention of heart disease as well.

So, how many vegetables have you eaten this week? Not enough? Become a vegetarian for one day a week and make a great start to healthier eating.

Feed the Muscles

It is important to fuel the muscles properly to be able to work out at a high intensity. The foods you choose to fuel your muscles also play an important role in allowing you to avoid injuries. So whether your goal is to tone up, get strong, gain muscle, heal from an injury, or participate in a sports activity, you need to feed your muscles.

Many people think that if they eat lots of protein, they'll get lean and strong, and build muscle. But it's the carbohydrates that we eat that give us the energy to use the protein we eat to build muscle. Those who participate in endurance sports, such as running and cycling, know the importance of eating a diet high in carbohydrates with some extra protein. But carbs are the foundation of performance, whether it's a tennis game, an aerobic workout, a golf game, or a bodybuilding routine.

Here is a list of good carbohydrate choices:

Legumes. Legumes are powerful energy foods, with vitamins and minerals in almost equal proportion to protein. They are a great meat alternative. Eat these at dinner the night before a morning workout.

Oatmeal. Oatmeal is a great stick-to-the-ribs energy food, full of vitamins and minerals with heart-health benefits (not just a slogan, but scientifically proven). Eat some oatmeal two to three hours before a workout.

Yogurt. Loaded with nutrients, such as bone-building calcium, protein, B vitamins, and the healthy immune-boosting bacteria that line our gastrointestinal tract. A great food, snack or snack topping, it's portable and easy to find. Eat a cup one hour before a workout to give you energy, especially when your last meal was a few hours before.

Bananas. Loaded with potassium and vitamin C, bananas fulfill the craving for both sweet and starch, and they are also versatile. Satisfy the urge for starch by adding them to a fruit salad or cereal, use them to thicken up a smoothie, stuff one in a bag to go, eat one on the run. Eat thirty minutes to an hour before a workout.

Salad with veggies. Veggies are loaded with vitamins, minerals, phytochemicals, and great complex carbohydrates. They fill us up without filling us out and they supply great energy. Add steamed or grilled vegetables to a $1/2$-cup cooked chilled pasta and make it a dinner salad.

Baked potato. Take a cue from bodybuilders who live on baked potatoes during their carb-eating training days. Make it a meal by adding legumes, salsa, or even cottage cheese.

High-fiber cereal. Start the day with a high-fiber wheat cereal with low-fat milk and a favorite fruit. Aside from the high-fiber benefits, whole grains supply energy you need to start the day, physically and mentally. Want to snack during the day? Put mixed high-fiber cereals in a baggie with dried fruit and munch away an hour or two before a workout.

These are just a few good choices of carbohydrate foods. So, if you want to look good, feel energetic, and perform well, feed your muscles.

Here are a few more ways to feed your muscles:

- **Eat often enough.** When you restrict your calories too much over a specified period, you send a signal to your body that a famine is coming. The body may then adjust your metabolic rate to slow down to conserve calories. The result? Most likely less strength, less energy, and even higher body fat.

- **Eat carbohydrates.** When you eat enough carbohydrates, you give your muscles the fuel to work out hard. This, in turn, gives your body the need to utilize all that protein you're taking in to make more muscle. Carbohydrates also feed your brain; when your blood sugar level is low from not eating enough carbs, your energy, focus, and performance are impaired. When you're in short supply of carbs, the process of turning protein into fuel for your muscles and brain is costly: it might impair performance, health, and the ability to lose weight and to build and repair your muscles. High-protein diets can also cause dehydration.

- **Drink water.** Water is stored in muscles with carbohydrates. This is the energy source for muscles. When you need to produce energy, the stored carbohydrates are used and water is released during the process. You need water to make and release energy. Guess what happens when you're dehydrated? You get fatigued easily. Water promotes stamina and performance, and helps to ward off those muscle cramps during intense exercise.

- **Eat a balanced diet.** If you eat lots of protein, you also need to eat enough fruits, veggies, and grains. And for vegetarians, it is important to get enough protein, iron, calcium, B_{12}, and vitamin D. Supplements, sports bars, and sports drinks are not a substitute for real food.

- **Eat wisely.** Be choosy about what kind of calories you eat. If I want to have energy for a tough workout, I choose a nutrient-dense food over a junk food. Of course, there is always room for a little junk— I recommend that you consume no more than 10 percent of your total daily calories in junk food (that's about 200 calories for most of us).

Not All Fats Are Created Equal

A fat is a fat when we refer to calories, but not all fats are equal when we refer to how they impact our health. The two main categories of dietary fats are saturated and unsaturated. It is estimated that fats make up at least 34 percent of the American diet, and the proportion of saturated fats to unsaturated is too high. Most of us are aware that saturated fats are the bad guys. These are the fats from animal sources, such as red meat, chicken, whole milk, and butter. Saturated fats are known for clogging arteries, leading to heart disease.

Unsaturated fats are divided into monounsaturated fats and polyunsaturated fats. Studies on these fats reveal that they have many health benefits. They are found in vegetables and legumes, such as corn, soybeans, and olives, along with oils, such as olive and canola oils (these are monounsaturated oils). Fish, such as salmon, are high in polyunsaturated fats, which are the best source of omega-3 fatty acids. All dietary fats contain both saturated and unsaturated fatty acids; it's just that the proportion of fatty acid type varies from food to food. For example, dairy products contain mostly saturated fat, but they also contain small amounts of monounsaturated and polyunsaturated fatty acids.

The least understood fats seem to be the trans fatty acids, formed during the hydrogenation process. These fats have been associated with an increase in cardiovascular disease and cancer as well as other chronic diseases. Trans fats are formed when we take polyunsaturated oils, such as corn oil, safflower oil, or any other vegetable oil, and chemically alter them from a liquid state to a more solid state (creating margarine or shortening). These polyunsaturated oils in a more solid state are then used in all those tasty baked goods (cookies, cakes, etc.) and for deep-frying.

Then there are the tropical fats: palm oil and coconut oil. While these are plant fats, they also happen to contain a high amount of saturated fatty acids, so they are considered a saturated fat. Unlike animal fats, which are solid at room temperature, these are liquid, so they can be used when a liquid fat is needed for flavor (such as movie popcorn). Don't be fooled by labels that read *no trans-fat* or *no partially hydrogenated fats*. These tropical fats are not healthy choices.

Fat is a necessary nutrient for all mammals, and scientists believe that our ability to store it contributed to the survival of our prehistoric ancestors. In fact, the Paleolithic diet is thought to have been rich in marine fat and the plant fats high in omega-3 fatty acids, while our modern diet is much richer in fat from animal sources (saturated) and more of the vegetable sources that contain omega-6 fatty acids. The greater availability of omega-3 fatty acids back in prehistoric days may have allowed humans to develop a complex brain and neural system.

So which fats should you eat? Eat more foods that contain polyunsaturated omega-3 fatty acids, including coldwater fish, such as salmon, shellfish, sardines, and mackerel. Some of the best vegetable sources are ground flaxseed, soybean products and soybean oils, and green leafy vegetables. A few monounsaturated fats are found in olive oil, canola oil, avocados, and nuts and seeds. Start by becoming a vegetarian for at least one day a week and include fish in your diet more often.

Alcohol, the Liquid Fat

Drinking alcohol is like eating liquid fat, and worse—it's fatter than fat! Fat contains nine calories per gram while alcohol contains seven. However, alcohol does not go through the exact same digestive process as fat. Your body uses energy to digest and absorb all nutrients, including fat, which means that about 10 percent of calories are used up during the digestive process. But that's not the case with alcohol. Alcohol begins to enter the bloodstream through the tongue, then the stomach (especially when it's empty), and then the remainder goes through the usual route of digestion and absorption through the small intestine. Even water doesn't reach the bloodstream and cells as quickly. So the calories in alcohol are just like "net fat calories" after digestion. Also, alcohol sugar is more easily stored as fat.

To make matters worse, if we start with a drink before eating, we're likely to eat and drink more than we intend to. How can we moderate our consumption of alcohol?

- Don't save up for the party. Eat often during the day—eat small, but eat.

- Eat a small snack an hour before the party. Don't have that first drink on an empty stomach, and try to eat something high in protein. Alcohol will enter the bloodstream faster on an empty stomach.

- Eat a piece of cheese or an appetizer with your first drink.

- Drink lots of water all day even if you're not thirsty and drink a few sips in between each drink. Alcohol will cause dehydration and fatigue the next day. Drinking water helps to compensate for that.

- Order a spicy Bloody Mary. Tomato juice is healthier; it can take the edge off your appetite and slow down how fast the alcohol is absorbed.

- Make smart trade-offs. A small glass of wine (4–5 oz.) will equal one shot (1 oz.) of hard liquor, calorie-wise, so consider this when making choices. Choose club soda instead of tonic (tonic is high in calories), and consider mixing hard liquor with club soda instead of straight up, since it'll last longer.

Water, a Top Nutrient

Yes, water is a nutrient, just like carbohydrates, fats, vitamins, and minerals, and if I were to list the top five healthy things you could do for yourself this year, drinking more water would definitely make the list. While most of us know that water is important, many of us tend to have difficulty drinking enough of it. But like all other healthy habits, drinking more water takes practice.

Interestingly, studies have found that those who drink more water tend to eat less. One study concluded that water drinkers ate almost 200 calories a day less than nonwater drinkers (*Water and Food Consumption Patterns of U.S. Adults from 1999–2001*, the North American Association for the Study of Obesity). Over the course of just one year, if you saved 200 calories a day, that could amount to a twenty-pound weight loss. Another study found that water consumers drank fewer soft drinks and generally followed healthier eating patterns.

Here's why water is so crucial to our health:

- Water in our blood forms the plasma that carries all vital nutrients to every cell in the body.

- Water in our urine and feces carries waste products out of the body. One major reason for constipation is dehydration.

- Water in our sweat releases heat through our skin, helping to maintain internal body temperature.

- Water plays a fundamental role in the transmission of our nervous system's electrical impulses.

- Water helps to dissolve and digest nutrients.

- Water promotes the biochemical reactions in our body, including the production and release of energy.

- Water in fluids surrounds our joints, providing lubrication and mobility.

Now that we know that water is one of the most important nutrients in our body, and that our body uses it for every biological function, how about we start drinking more, little by little? I keep a small water bottle with me at all times. This seems to help, even when I'm at home. Who knows, it might become a habit.

A few tips about water and sports nutrition:

- Dehydration is one of the most common reasons for fatigue during exercise and a common reason for fatigue in general.

- Starting to drink water at the beginning of an exercise session may be too late.

- Exercising less than ninety minutes? Water is most likely all you need as long as you've eaten food within the last hour or so.

- Cool water is absorbed faster into our bloodstream than water at room temperature.

- Drinking water does not cause water retention.

- Thirst is not a good indicator of water or fluid needs.

- Children and older adults do not have as acute a thirst mechanism as healthy adults.

During the summer you need to drink more water, especially if you're exercising in hot humid weather. When the humidity is high, the body uses more water to keep the core body temperature down. Here are some tips for drinking water when you exercise:

- Drink two cups (on average) one hour prior to exercise (up to one quart may be consumed one hour pre-exercise for more intense sessions).

- Drink half a cup every fifteen minutes during exercise.

- Weigh yourself periodically before and after exercise. If you are hydrated and drinking enough water, your weight doesn't change. If you've lost weight after your exercise session, then you haven't taken in enough water for optimum performance.

- The water you drink should be cool, not room temperature. Cool water empties from the stomach faster, reaching your bloodstream and cells faster.

- Drink a low-carbohydrate sports drink if your exercise will exceed ninety minutes.

Some of the signs that may mean you're not getting enough water are mild headaches, feeling cold, dry mouth, faster heart rate than usual during exercise, and even nausea. If you're hitting the links, but you didn't eat breakfast and you're planning to be on the course for four hours, let's say, a good idea is to mix Gatorade with water and drink that before the start of the round.

It is recommended that we drink eight glasses of water a day. But what many of us don't realize is that we may need to drink even more than that to compensate for dehydration caused by other things. For example:

- Drink coffee? Add one cup of water for every cup of coffee you drink.

- Drink tea other than herbal? Add half a cup of water for every cup of tea you drink.

- Drink soda with caffeine (this includes both diet and regular)? Add a cup of water for every ten to twelve ounces of soda you drink.

- Did you drink alcohol last night? Yep, add another cup of water for every drink.

- Exercised for one hour? Add at least two cups of water for even moderate/light exercise. Longer or more intense exercise requires more water. More water is required for outdoor exercise or exercise that is prolonged (hiking, or endurance events, for example).

Do you eat very few fresh fruits and raw veggies? Eight glasses is the general guideline if you're taking in foods with medium to high water content and other fluids, such as milk, juice, soups, and so on. Are you on a high-protein diet with few or no carbs? If so, you need extra water, too, since your kidneys have to work a bit harder flushing out unusable protein molecules. Are you taking medications? Your kidneys filter out the metabolic products of medications, so your kidneys will function better with extra water. Some medications may require more water than usual, so check with your doctor. Do you have cardiovascular disease, such as high blood pressure? Extra water is especially important—extra water will keep the blood flowing more easily (it helps reduce viscosity, or blood thickness).

Tips to Help Lose Weight

Keep a food journal. Write down what and when you eat throughout a day and why you ate what you did when. The journal will help you become aware of what you eat and your eating patterns. You tend to gain weight when you eat for entertainment, comfort, or stress reduction.

Become aware of meal timing. Eating earlier in the day prevents you from getting too hungry, losing control, and overeating in the evening.

Learn your calorie budget. Know how much you can eat and still lose weight so you can be sure to fuel your body with an adequate amount of essential nutrients.

Eat slowly. The brain needs about twenty minutes to receive the signal that you've eaten your fill. Practice by putting your fork down between bites and taking pauses throughout the meal.

Keep away from food sources that tempt you. Out of sight, out of mind, out of mouth. Hide high-calorie foods and keep healthy snacks readily available.

Taste your food. Calories should be tasted, not wasted. Do nothing else while eating and really savor your food.

Stick to your shopping list. Always bring a food list when grocery shopping and never shop while you're hungry.

Buy individually wrapped packages. Buy your favorite snack foods in individual serving sizes to avoid overeating and further temptation.

Set realistic goals. Weight loss greater than 1 percent of your body weight for over two weeks can be dangerous—you can lose muscle, including cardiac muscle. Aim to lose half a pound to two pounds a week to ensure that you are losing body fat.

Foods to Avoid

Movie theater popcorn—with butter, 1,640 calories and 126 g fat (73 g saturated)

Prime rib—16 oz. contains 1,280 calories and 94 g fat (52 g saturated)

Cheese—1 oz. contains 100 calories and 9 g fat (6 g saturated)

Pizza—Domino's Hand Tossed Cheese ($1/8$ pie)—250 calories and 7 g fat (4 g saturated)

General Tso's chicken—1,600 calories and 59 g fat (11 g saturated)

Hamburgers—6 oz. burger on a bun contains 660 calories and 36 g fat (17 g saturated)

Doughnuts—an old-fashioned doughnut has 250 calories and 15 g fat (3 g saturated)

Cinnamon rolls—670 calories and 34 g fat (14 g saturated)

Croissants—5 oz. almond croissant contains 630 calories and 42 g fat (18 g saturated)

French fries—large order contains 500 calories and 28 g fat (13 g saturated fat)

Tortilla chips—a basket (51 chips) contains 640 calories and 34 g fat (6 g saturated)

Calorie Intake* by Age and Activity Level

MALES				FEMALES			
ACTIVITY LEVEL	SEDENTARY*	MOD. ACTIVE	ACTIVE	ACTIVITY LEVEL	SEDENTARY	MOD. ACTIVE	ACTIVE
AGE				AGE			
16	2400	2800	3200	16	1800	2000	2400
17	2400	2800	3200	17	1800	2000	2400
18	2400	2800	3200	18	1800	2000	2400
19–20	2600	2800	3000	19–20	2000	2200	2400
21–25	2400	2800	3000	21–25	2000	2200	2400
26–30	2400	2600	3000	26–30	1800	2000	2400
31–35	2400	2600	3000	31–35	1800	2000	2200
36–40	2400	2600	2800	36–40	1800	2000	2200
41–45	2200	2600	2800	41–45	1800	2000	2200
46–50	2200	2400	2800	46–50	1800	2000	2200
51–55	2200	2400	2800	51–55	1600	1800	2200
56–60	2200	2400	2600	56–60	1600	1800	2200
61–65	2000	2400	2600	61–65	1600	1800	2000
66–70	2000	2200	2600	66–70	1600	1800	2000
71–75	2000	2200	2600	71–75	1600	1800	2000
76 and up	2000	2000	2400	76 and up	1600	1800	2000

*Calorie levels are based on the Estimated Energy Requirements (EER) and activity levels from the Institute of Medicine Dietary Reference *Intakes Macro Nutrients Report*, 2002.

Sedentary = less than 30 minutes a day of moderate physical activity in addition to daily activities.
Moderately Active = at least 30 minutes up to 60 minutes a day of moderate physical activity in addition to daily activities.
Active = 60 or more minutes a day of moderate physical activity in addition to daily activities.

Source website: http://www.mypyramid.gov/professionals/pdf_calorie_levels.html

Grilled cheese sandwich—500 calories and 33 g fat (17 g saturated fat)

Fettuccine Alfredo—1,500 calories and 97 g fat (48 g saturated)

Starbucks white chocolate mocha (made with whole milk)—600 calories and 25 g fat (15 g saturated)

Pancakes with syrup and margarine—3 pancakes with 1/4-cup syrup and 1 tablespoon margarine contain 770 calories and 22 g fat (9 g saturated)

Portion Sizes—Bigger Is Not Better

One of the most important factors for weight-loss success is understanding the need to control portion sizes. Even if a meal exceeds the recommended amount of fat, you can compensate by reducing your portion size.

Many people underestimate how fast calories add up (especially when you're celebrating!). So here are some portion sizes to eat by:

- Meat, red or that so-called white meat (pork): 1 serving (3 ounces) is about the size of a deck of cards
- Baked potato: 1 serving, the size of a computer mouse
- Rice: 1 serving, about the size of a golf ball
- Pasta: 1 serving, about 1/2 tennis ball
- Steamed vegetables: who cares
- Fish, such as sole, red snapper, or mahi mahi: 1 serving is equal to 3 ounces; however, double the deck of cards since most fish is lighter in weight
- Butter: 1 serving, the size of a small thumbnail (the nail, not the whole thumb)
- Cheese: the size of a pair of dice

- Muffin: you don't want to know! Okay, slightly bigger than a golf ball (All kidding aside, that average 5 oz. low-fat muffin contains about 70 calories an ounce and that's without the added fat and sugar)

In general, smaller is better. Think about the quality of the food, not the quantity. Eating slowly and focusing on taste can help create a more satisfying experience. Eating before you are hungry can help you reduce the portions you consume, too.

Snacking for Health and Energy

Healthy eating and high energy go hand in hand. Snacking can help you feel more energetic and think more clearly. Snacking often can improve your mood, boost your energy, and help curb cravings. Every time you eat, your body acts like a furnace, raising your metabolism. You actually burn more calories when you eat more often, if you take in the same number of calories in total for the day. When you start snacking more often, you usually eat less at each meal.

What should we snack on? My philosophy is that any food can be a snack, and any snack can be a minimeal. Snacks are small portions of foods we usually have as meals.

The Lean Grill

You can significantly reduce your fat intake when you choose to grill lean. Start with grilled shrimp or lobster and add gazpacho or a large salad. Shellfish is low in fat and calories. Prepare the food with a nonfat marinade. Grill up lots of veggies for side dishes. Peppers, zucchini, eggplant, onions, tomatoes, and corn on the cob are all healthy, tasty choices when you grill them using a nonfat butter spray.

Grill fish. Even a high-fat fish is healthier than meat because it contains less saturated and total fat than red meat. When you do grill meat, grill lean cuts. Choose leaner cuts, such as top round, tenderloin, flank steak, and chicken breasts. Marinade them in advance, using fruits such as limes and kiwi to tenderize them.

If you are thinking of starting a diet or a specific eating plan of any kind, make sure it is safe and one that you can keep up with and follow today, next month, and next year. If you don't see yourself being able to do it forever, don't even think of starting it because when you go off it (and, believe me, you will), you'll gain the weight back, plus more.

Hopefully, these tips will help you eat for better health. Combined with the exercises in this book, you should be well on your way to improving your golf game.

Putting It Together

Golf is a challenging sport, a diverting pastime, and a fantastic excuse to spend a beautiful day outdoors. But like most things in life, golf is far more rewarding if you are in top physical shape. By following one of the fitness routines outlined in this book, and by observing good eating habits, I guarantee that a whole new world of accomplishment will open up to you, on the links and off. You will not only be improving your golf game, you will enjoy increased energy levels and find it far easier to mentally focus, whether you are facing a long drive to a distant green or a personal or work-related challenge.

Whether you are trying to lose weight, improve your stamina, or simply put on more muscle, the exercises in *Fit to a Tee* will help you accomplish your goals, specifically with an eye toward improving your golf game. And once you experience the difference these exercises can make to your game and to the quality of your life, you will find it easier and easier to continue training year-round. Take it from a life-long golfer and fitness professional like me: stick with one of my fitness routines and soon enough, you'll be fit to a tee!

Contact Information

If you have a question on fitness and exercise for golf, or on general fitness,
you may write, email, or call us:
Attention: Edward Jackowski, Ph.D.
Exude Fitness
1275 First Avenue, Suite 283
Web address: www.exude.com
Email address: Edward@exude.com
Telephone: 212-644-9559

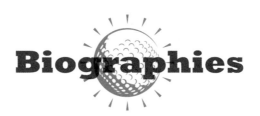

Biographies

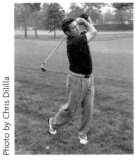

Photo by Chris Dililla

Edward Jackowski, Ph.D., has been a professional in the fitness industry for over twenty years. In 1985, he created an innovative fitness company, called EXUDE, which has become one of the most successful fitness companies in the country. Headquartered in Manhattan, EXUDE offers one-on-one training services throughout New York City, the Tri-State, and southern California.

Edward has written a number of books, including *America, You're Exercising Wrong*; *Hold it! You're Exercising Wrong*; *Escape Your Shape*; *Escape Your Weight*; and *Jump into Fitness*. He was the first fitness advisor and fitness columnist for AARP's *Modern Maturity* magazine, and has written for a myriad of publications and websites, including the *Daily News*, *Salute* magazine (for the United States armed forces), *WebMd*, and others. Edward has been interviewed one on one by Barbara Walters, Diane Sawyer, and Pat Robertson, and is currently one of *Star* magazine's lifestyle/fitness contributing advisors. He also writes a lifestyle and fitness column for *Healthy Living NYC* magazine.

Over the years, Edward has developed and taught fitness programming for children, the elderly, business people with hectic lifestyles, the physically challenged, frustrated

exercisers, and athletes. Edward also volunteers his time with the American Diabetes Association (ADA), educating young people and the elderly on the importance of exercise, and he is a board member for the Youth Health Coalition and the Neuropathy Foundation/Charcot-Marie Tooth. In 2002, Edward was selected as Avon's Fitness Guru of the Year. In 2004, ZonePerfect Bars enlisted Edward's expertise, in conjunction with SELF magazine's Workout in the Park series, to help women across the country exercise to lower their risk of breast cancer.

Edward holds a B.B.A. from Baruch Business College and an M.A. and doctorate in behavioral management from International University. Edward is a professional member of the American College of Sports Medicine and IDEA, and is nationally certified by the Aerobics and Fitness Association of America in both aerobic conditioning and personal training. To contact Edward, please email him at Info@exude.com.

Doug Mauch is a PGA Member Class A-1 Professional who has been teaching golf since 1990, when he turned pro and started his career at Westchester Country Club in Rye, New York. Doug was a teaching pro at Ardsley Country Club in Westchester, New York, for three years and then at the Maidstone Club in East Hampton, New York. He spent 1996–1997 at the Augusta National Golf Club, home of the Masters. From 1997 through 2002, Doug became the head golf pro at Tradition Golf Club in La Quinta,

California, the West Coast home of Arnold Palmer, where Doug personally instructed Arnold, making him one of the few pros to have taught Arnold Palmer, since Arnold worked with his father.

Doug was president of the MET PGA Assistants Association in 1994–1995 and was a member of the MET PGA's Assistant Squire Cup Team in 1994, 1995, and 1996. In 2002, Doug won the Callaway Golf Invitational and in 2003, he was named Callaway's Golf Club Fitter of the year. In 2005, Doug was elected to the MET PGA Board of Directors and for the past three years he has been the head professional at Wheatley Hills Golf Club in East Williston, New York.

Doug is sponsored by Callaway Golf and is a master staff professional for Callaway Golf. Doug graduated from Molloy College in Rockville Centre, New York, where he received his B.A. in business administration. He and his wife Meghan have two small children, Connor and Malloy Mae. They live on Long Island, New York. If you would like to contact Doug, email him at Dougmauch@aol.com

Cindy Jennings (C.J.) Reeves is a Class A Member of the LPGA Teaching Division and a PGA Member, and is considered one of the Northeast's premier teaching and swing coaches. C.J. was named a "Top 50 Instructor" by Golf for Women magazine in 2001 and 2003–2005. In 2001, she was the first woman to receive the Metropolitan PGA Teacher of the Year Award.

C.J. won the PGA Women's Stroke Play in 2005 and the MET PGA Women's Match Play in 2002. In 1998 and 2000, she won the LPGA Northeast Section Championship and represented the Northeast in the 1999 and 2001 McDonald's Championship, an LPGA major.

C.J. attended Rollins College in Winter Park, Florida, on a golf scholarship and graduated with a B.A. in business administration. She currently teaches at Century Country Club in Purchase, New York, and is affiliated with the TaylorMade Golf Company. She is married to John Reeves, head professional at Willow Ridge Country Club in Harrison, New York. They have a six-year-old son, Justin, and reside in Bedford, New York. If you would like to contact C.J., email her at cjreeves12@msn.com.

Adrian Fryer is a PGA Professional, Class AA. More than twenty-five years of teaching experience has enabled Adrian to accurately diagnose swing flaws and offer practical advice for the beginners, club golfers, professionals, and national players he coaches. Adrian was instrumental in launching Drivetime Golf Center in 1991 in Warrington, England, which today is a thriving center for golf coaching and instruction. Adrian's instruction ideas have been featured in *Golf World* magazine and, in 2002, he was hand-picked as swing coach for the new TEAM TG instruction series for Britain's monthly golf magazine *Today's Golfer*. He is currently a regular contributor to *Today's Golfer*.

Adrian has had years of coaching experience, including coaching the Cheshire County Ladies' Golf Association, as coach to Cheshire County Boys Champion, Ladies County Champion, and Girls Champion, England U 18's boys and schoolboy team members, and English Girls and Boys team members, as well as coaching the two-time winner and British PGA National Assistants Champion. In addition, Adrian was the organizer of three North Region PGA teaching conferences, featuring Pete Cowen (coach to Lee Westwood, Darren Clarke, and others), Denis Pugh (coach to Colin Montgomerie and others), and John Jacobs OBE, former Ryder Cup captain and world-renowned coach. Adrian currently provides Inner Game workshops alongside sports psychologist Dr. Karl Morris (mental coach to Darren Clarke, Paul McGinley, Graeme McDowell, and the England cricket team).

Adrian is also an inventor of several training aids aimed at improving swing flaws for players of all levels, including the patented SWINGMATIC (www.stopmyslice.com).

Adrian has four children and in lives in Warrington, England. To contact Adrian, email him at adrian@adrianfryergolf.com.

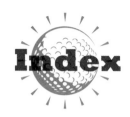

Index

F

W